How Angels Die

A CONFESSION

by Guy Blews

Published by Waldorf Publishing

2140 Hall Johnson Road
#102-113
Grapevine, Texas 76051

www.WaldorfPublishing.com

How Angels Die: A Confession by Guy Blews
ISBN 9781634439374

Library of Congress Control Number: 2014948138
Copyright Guy Blews © 2014

Movie Reviews for "37: A Final Promise"

"Randall Batinkoff delivers an affecting and involving romantic drama"

"An old-fashioned tearjerker set to a goth-rock soundtrack"

"The leads are impressively adroit at keeping the film grounded in persuasive emotional truth"

"Batinkoff and Thompson develop a potent chemistry together"

- Variety

"An incredible love story based on actual events"

- Huffington Post

"Love this movie! A modern day 'Love Story'... the epitome of being in love"

- UBN Radio

"Batinkoff handles his directing and acting abilities quite well"

- The Examiner

How Angels Die - A Confession

Foreword

I met Guy Blews at a club called The Mint on Pico Boulevard in Los Angeles well over a decade ago. He was thirty-five at the time and the lead singer of a rock band. Of course, he had the requisite pretty girlfriend by his side.

His upper body was riddled with tattoos; one of them, the number 37 on his left arm, particularly caught my attention. When I asked him what it stood for, he smiled and told me it was the age he was going to die. When I questioned how he knew that, he said, "Because I'm going to do it myself." I was intrigued - and this was how our friendship began.

I would see Guy and his girlfriend once in a while. After some months and many questions, I learned that Guy's 'expiration date' was associated with witnessing his innocent younger brother being ravaged and killed by a horrible disease.

It devastated Guy that life could be so cruel and the world did not stop to care.

As a result, he did not ascribe to the preciousness of life because he saw how easily and without consequence it could be taken. His plan was to get out of this world at thirty-seven, before anything bad could happen to him.

I did everything in my power to try to talk him out of it, but he laughed at my attempts and told me nothing would change his mind. He was thirty-six when we lost touch, but the question always lingered: what happened to Guy Blews and did he do what he said he would do?

Two years later, I walked into Gold's Gym in Venice, California and saw Guy - you can only imagine my great surprise. I was happy and relieved to see him. When I asked how old he was, he told me he was thirty-eight. My brow furrowed - he had not followed through with his plan. And his girlfriend? How was she? He told me she died. When I asked him how, he replied, "She killed herself."

He then recounted the story that you will read in this book. It is a harrowing love story which is both tragic and beautiful. It forces you to think about things you may never have considered before - like what you would do if the person you loved most in the world wanted to die and asked you to help them do it.

It also asks you to confront your own mortality and a person's choice concerning end of life decisions. One day, we will all be confronted with this reality.

How Angels Die - A Confession

This is the story of two people, on very different paths in life, who manage to help each other confront an unimaginable situation - a devastating tale of unconditional love which so shocked and moved me that I spent many years developing it and adapting it into a movie named "37: A Final Promise" which is now in theaters and on VOD everywhere.

We took the liberty of changing some details in the film because they were simply too graphic and painful.

Here is the real story.

Randall Batinkoff
August 2014

How Angels Die - A Confession

Author's Note

Due to the nature of this book and the law in the United States, I have changed the names of those involved in order to protect them against a justice system that I feel is beyond acceptable in its reach and power.

I allowed this story to be released as I feel it gives a clear message of love, compassion and choice that might assist others in their ability to understand that our society is not easily divided into right and wrong, that life is fraught with fragility, and that we should all have the final say in how our lives might end.

I believe very strongly the publication of this book would have been Jemma's wish. I struggle everyday with the fact she had to endure so much against her will because of a system that, hypocritically, will not allow each of us fundamental choices regarding life and liberty.

I hope our story will encourage a more open-minded outlook on the right to die and all that it allows, accepts or prevents.

I had been balancing on the precipice of discovery for two full days; waiting, agonized, for the right time to find her. I am still not quite sure how clear my thought process was at the time. There was trepidation for certain, a little fear, a sense of duty and even a form of hope that it was, at last, done.

I was certainly on some form of auto-pilot as I opened the door to her ground floor Hollywood apartment. Despite what she had said to me the last time we spoke, I still did not want to admit to myself what I knew I was about to see and more importantly what I knew I had lost.

The door opened into a sunlit filled sitting room that looked through a bay window onto the street outside. The back of the antique-looking brown leather sofa was a few feet away and the coffee table had the remote controls from the TV lying haphazardly next to an empty bottle of Snapple with a purple straw standing proudly in it. The cushion on the sofa still held the indentation of her shoulders and head from where she used to lie watching endless television shows until she fell asleep. I stepped inside and instantly felt the lifelessness of the apartment as I scanned the area in front of me to see if she was there. She was not.

My eyes drifted slightly forward and to the left at the archway that led into the galley kitchen. I called out, dreading a reply.

- Angel?

Nothing.

A vacuum of silence in the apartment.

Outside, through the sheer curtains, I could sense the cars whisking down the hill making the most of the shortcut that took them to Melrose Avenue a block and a half away. I paused.

I summoned up the courage to walk past the square dining room table. The love note I had written her was still there; I looked through the archway into the kitchen. Empty. I was now at one end of the short corridor that had a bathroom to the right, a spare bedroom ahead, and her bedroom door on the far left. I stopped.

I knew where she was, but I had to gather the nerve to move again, towards something I did not want to believe.

- Angel?

How Angels Die - A Confession

Silence.

I took three more steps and looked to my right, into the bathroom. Everything seemed in order, but I knew that it was not, I knew there was something dreadful waiting for me. I was hesitant now. Afraid.

I paused for a split second before taking a final step towards the bedroom on the left, her bedroom. I slowly raised my eyes, expanding my field of vision. I could see the tall palm plant in the corner, the foot of the bed, the ruffled cream sheets, her feet, motionless, there, relaxed. The stillness crept over me as I somehow, somehow found the courage to step into the room. I moved forward, I looked to the right and there she was, My Angel.

I had last seen her at seven o'clock on Saturday morning -

The early light was seeping through the slats of the wooden blinds at the head of the bed onto the white tops of the small, brown-tinted plastic tubes that held the sleeping pills. They were standing on the Moroccan bedside table like misplaced toy soldiers, stationary, nestled amongst the telephone, the digital alarm clock, a pair of discarded earrings, an unread book, and the simple glass vase that held some healthy green bamboo shoots with a few sprouting leaves. There was also a freshly poured long-stemmed glass of wine, alone and out of place.

She had sat on her side of the bed, her legs dangling over the edge like those of a little girl, weakly resisting bedtime before submitting to the inevitable.

As she leaned across to grab the three plastic containers, she looked at me, deliberately avoiding eye contact with what her hand was reaching for and eventually found.

How Angels Die - A Confession

- I don't want to say goodbye this time - She said.

I was crouched in front of her with my hands resting tenderly on her knees, looking up, not uttering a word. Her eyes avoided mine as she loosened the white tops and emptied out a handful of pills before picking up the glass of wine - the nectar that would ease the consumption of the poison. She managed to swallow five mouthfuls of the little multi-colored specks, washing them down with uncertain gulps.

I watched. I did not speak; I did not move. I was too full of dread to do either - too empty to object.

Within minutes she was drowsy and losing consciousness; she tried to maneuver herself into a lying position, but these days she was weak and helpless. On occasion, I would have to carry her to the bathroom because she could no longer walk unaided, and the difficulty she encountered with any form of movement was a constant reminder of how much she did not want to be here anymore.

Now, I engaged my body to help.

I stood up and leaned over her so that I could gently ease her into a comfortable position - a soft pillow under her head, a sheet over her legs.

She lay there, on her side, with sinking, heavy eyelids, looking at me.

How Angels Die - A Confession

- I love you... I love you... I love you...

She kept saying it. Over and over.

I settled down next to her. I lay on my side, facing her, tears filling my eyes as I looked unwaveringly at My Beautiful Angel - her dark brown hair fell around her pretty face with her high cheekbones and her full, soft lips, her little button nose and her perfect eyebrows. She was slipping away and I knew that I only had a few moments left with her.

- I love you too, My Angel, so much... So very much.

I am not sure she heard me, or if she felt me put my hand softly on her face as I stroked her to sleep. I hope she did. Her eyes fluttered erratically until they closed and then her breathing slowed until she barely moved. I lay there, motionless, helpless, watching over her as she gently expired before my eyes; my sad, heavy eyes that drifted from her face to her chest to see if she would, at last, be still.

My heart beat slowly, but with power. I could feel the tension rise from the pit of my stomach into my throat as I was totally immersed in these final, lingering minutes. I wanted to stay there all day to guard over her, protect her as she left this cruel world and floated to a more peaceful place. The place she longed to be. The place she had sought out for so many months.

How Angels Die - A Confession

Was she there yet? Had she begun her journey? Was she aware that she was leaving?

My body became slightly numb and the tips of my fingers cooled as I watched her become more and more peaceful. I felt myself fill with an indescribable sickness, yet I still felt empty. I was heartbroken, the intensity of the situation crushed me inside. The truth of losing her crushed my entire existence in some way, but I was compelled to stay as long as I felt able. I would wait until she was, I thought, dead, or at least as near death as she could be. I was not sure, but I thought her breathing would just slow down until it stopped and then she would be gone. It would be over. She would be released.

I do not know how long I lay there, focusing on her. I was meandering within the parameters of emotional pain and a kind of practical martyrdom. There was a part of me that wanted to shake her, wake her from her never-ending slumber, bring her back to life; but the stronger part of me resisted this urge. This was the part that was resigned to letting her go, allowing her to evaporate in the most inconspicuous way possible, without fanfare, without consent, without anyone knowing until it was too late.

At some stage, I thought, I will have to force myself to leave. I felt as if she would not be able to complete her final journey if I was there. My being there might hold her back, keep her from expiring completely, act as an anchor that is attached to the chord of life and will not allow her to drift off into the eternal darkness. I had to leave in order that I might set her free from that which she could no longer bear to face.

I also had to leave so that I would not be implicated in her death. And here lay my biggest dilemma; this abandonment was my one area of weakness. How would I be able to live with myself if I let her go - if I was the one to let her die? She had been so determined, so certain that she could not carry on "like this", and in her certainty I had, somehow, found the strength to be there for her, to support her no matter what the consequences might be.

She used to say

- What if they think you helped me? I don't want anything to happen to you because of me.

- Don't worry, Angel. I'll be fine. I'll be okay - I would always reply.

Despite my easy words, I was unfamiliar with the severity of being present at the outset of a suicide, and I was concerned that it could be very serious for me should the law single me out for blame, no matter how much I felt I was doing the right thing.

I had come to the point, the moment, where I could no longer linger in an oblivion of sadness, wishing I could hold her forever in a place with no pain, no fear, no hurt...

How Angels Die - A Confession

I could not stay with her indefinitely, I could no longer nestle up to her in the hope that it might not really be happening; I had to get up. I had to let go.

And so now, hesitantly, tenderly, for the last time, I kissed her on the lips. I had done the same every morning before I left her apartment for as long as we had been together. Her lips felt warm and soft, they were cushioned with love and I held myself there for a few seconds before separating; then I slowly moved my hand away from her face and slipped off the bed.

She had always let me kiss her without moving her lips, it was as if she was a life-size porcelain doll, waiting, unaware, for that perfect touch; and today was no different, despite her being more fragile now than ever before.

I took four or five careful steps away from the bed and then I turned to her. I stood for a few more seconds looking at her, absorbing her for the very last time, remembering her.

- I love you, My Angel. I love you... Goodbye - I whispered.

She did not stir. She was still. Very, very still. I finally turned away.

I walked quietly down the corridor towards the sitting room and, as I had always done, I wrote her a love note in the little square book she had left out on the wooden dining table the night before.

I love you, My Sweet Angel
With all my heart
XXXXX

I stared at the note, momentarily realizing that she would never see these words. I hoped they would be with her when she left, they would fly with her soul on her Angel wings.

She would know my love, wherever she may go.

I closed the apartment door behind me and carefully turned the key in the lock. I stood, lingering, with my hand on the doorknob. I was suffering now, internally, contemplating everything I was leaving behind, everything I was losing, everything I would never experience again. I kept persuading myself that I had no option but to leave, no matter how much I wanted to turn back; for her sake, for my sake. The hands of time were ticking and her destiny was waiting for her, beckoning, beyond my control.

At that moment, I felt that she was no longer mine.

3

Jemma and I had met just over seven years before; at a house party in Bel Air - it was a typical "LA" gathering filled with dolled up girls and men on a mission. As I walked aimlessly around the numerous rooms deciding where to settle, she had pointed at me from a huddle of people, saying

- And who are you?

I introduced myself. She stepped out of the huddle.

- I like your outfit - She stated.

- Outfit? - I laughed - Like a costume? I'm not a clown, you know.

I was a singer at the time, thirty years old. I had come to Los Angeles to play live concerts and record in studios; I was a singer with a purpose, and having designed clothes before moving to America, my image was very deliberate.

I was wearing a black fitted shirt and jeans, with leather boots and a sturdy belt. I am English, and therefore my look is slightly more European than most of the men in the USA. I am six feet tall and slim, I have most of my clothes tailored to a specific style, not necessarily a classically smart style, but they are made to fit me well. I also have numerous monotone black tattoos. My brown hair is cropped and slightly messy. I did not look like the other guests at the party who were in suits or slacks, which was probably why Jemma had picked on me. She was surrounded by four or five other people but she turned away from their conversation to grab my attention and she proceeded to question me.

- And how come you're here? You don't fit in at all - She continued.

- Thanks, I think - I replied - I was invited by a friend. You?

- This is my boss's party. I had to be here.

- Oh. I'm sorry. Does it hurt? - I teased.

- Not so much now - She said, smiling at me.

She reached forward and touched my arm, she looked at my tattoos that were visible below the slightly rolled up sleeve of my shirt, they stopped at my wrist but she probably guessed that they went all the way up to my shoulder.

- Do they hurt? - She inquired.

How Angels Die - A Confession

I looked down at my arm, her hand on my tattoos. I felt her gentle touch, it warmed me.

- Not right now - I said, quietly.

I wanted to lean forward and kiss her, hold her face in my hands, feel her closer to me. But no. I stood my ground.

- You're funny - She said.

- Funny haha or funny weird? - I asked.

She looked at me for a second and then smiled softly before speaking.

- I'm not sure...

We talked lightly for a few minutes, the words were unimportant but the attraction was unmistakable; she was confident in her approach and probing with her inquiries, unafraid to make herself the center of attention without seeming brash.

She was pretty, that was unquestionable, and she smiled often, displaying characterful, yet near-perfect white teeth that complimented her bright blue eyes. She was wearing high heels, sexy slim fit jeans and a top that was, I later found out, a silk scarf ingeniously fashioned to cover her front but reveal her smooth and tanned back.

I assumed she had a boyfriend; she was too lovely to be single and too at ease to be looking. After a few minutes of talking I made sure to make my excuses and leave her be. I did not want to seem too keen, and I surmised that I would stand out more if I walked away rather than appearing to hang around for too long like the other guys in the huddle.

- I better let you get back to your friends. It was good to meet you - I said - What's your name?

I took her hand with both of mine as I spoke.

- Jemma - She replied.

- Bye, Jemma - I said, before walking away.

Despite my cool exterior, I hoped that the meeting had been as powerful for her as it had been for me; I tried not to linger on the thought and moved further into the party.

I quickly found my friend, Charlie, who introduced me to some people that he knew, and I spent the rest of the evening in conversation; but these people did not engage me, how could they? I could not stop thinking about Jemma - my mind was working overtime on how to get her number.

All the while I was aware of where she was, carefully keeping my strategic distance before building up the courage to take the next step; if she had a boyfriend it would be the last step I took towards her and I would have to back away with as much honor as possible.

Being a guy is always fraught with the possibility of rejection, but if we do not ask we will never know, and that is far worse than the momentary sting we might receive from a brush off. Over the years we learn to walk away with dignity - or at least we think we do.

Before I left that night I made a point of talking to Jemma. She was outside, by the pool, dancing with one of the suit-guys at the edge of the raised wooden dance floor; I touched her lightly on the shoulder, she turned to see who it was, a smile lit up her face.

- I just wanted to say goodbye - I said.

- You should call me - She replied.

There, she had said it; she had saved me the trouble and the worry. No awkward questions or inquiries were necessary.

- I will - I said - What's your number?

- Do you have a pen? - She asked, looking at my hands to see if I happened to be carrying one.

- No - I replied, smiling - But I have a memory.

She laughed, as I hoped she would, and then she paused for a second before looking up at me and saying

- I work at the Photographic Art Gallery in Beverly Hills.

I smiled. Mission accomplished. That was all I needed. Jemma had craftily left it up to me to find the number. I did, that night, when I got to my house.

On my drive home, I had re-played the evening in my mind; the way she had stopped me whilst she was in the midst of a conversation with other people, her natural smile that seemed to fill the area around her with light, the simple yet sensual movement of her body when she danced, the slow motion of our goodbye, and the ease with which she turned back to her dancing partner after having told me to call her at work right in front of him. Everything about her appealed to me, and later, as I closed my eyes to drift off to sleep, a smile spread across my face. I felt mildly effervescent about the possibilities of Jemma.

I know there are many theories on when a man should call a woman - should he leave it for two days so as not to seem desperate? Or should he wait longer in the hope that she will think he has plenty of other options? I am not one for playing games, and judging by the way Jemma had approached me the previous night I figured she probably had little time for the typical routines either. I thought it would be best to make the unexpected move of calling the next day, which I did, as I stood in my little white house in Laguna, looking at the ocean through the French doors.

The receptionist put me on hold. I was on hold for a while. When Jemma finally came to the phone I said, or rather, I shouted

- Hello, Gorgeous!

She paused slightly, and then she said

- Can I call you back? What's your number?

Damn, I remember thinking to myself, I just managed to mess that one up and I only said two words. I gave her my number and never expected to hear from her again - although I did wait by the phone for the call back.

An hour or so later my phone rang; it was Jemma.

- I was in a meeting when you called - She said.

- Oh, good timing then - I replied.

- Yes - She laughed - Especially because everybody in the room heard you shout "Hello, Gorgeous!"

She said these last two words with an English accent, to push the point home. I began to laugh, hoping she would too. She did.

- So, did they give you a hard time?

- No - She said - I'm the boss's right hand man, so they can't really, but they all looked at me and I went bright red. It definitely made the meeting memorable, though.

She had an infectious giggle and an easy manner, she was interesting and interested, and best of all, she was clearly intrigued by me. Jemma later recalled thinking I was a little nutty, but she liked it. She asked plenty of questions and gave plenty of answers, she was open and forthright, and after twenty minutes we had built a rapport that would last for the rest of her life and would be with me for the rest of mine. I knew that she had something special, even then, but I could not quite put my finger on it. She was refreshing and zestful, she was calm and sensitive, she seemed to enjoy life yet she was not over-powering. She was incredibly endearing and I wanted to see her again.

- Would you like to have dinner on Sunday night? - I asked, finally.

- That would be great - She replied without hesitation.

Unfortunately, in my haste to see her again, I had forgotten a promise I had made to go backstage to an

How Angels Die - A Confession

Alanis Morrisette concert in Anaheim on the same night - I had double booked. I called to cancel with Jemma as soon as I realized my mistake.

- I am so sorry.

- That's okay - She said - You've just blown your one and only chance.

And then she burst into laughter and continued with

- Who's your date then?

- My buddy, Michael - I replied.

- Oh, it's like that is it?!

She was clearly mischievous, at ease with herself, and with me. I really wanted to miss the concert because I really wanted to spend time with Jemma, but I could not let Michael down and so Jemma and I made arrangements to meet up on the Tuesday night instead.

I picked her up from her apartment in Hollywood at 8PM, she was ready and waiting, which was rare for an LA girl. We went to Indochine on 3rd Street - I had chosen this restaurant because it was full of people in the scene so we could both enjoy the view and feel like we were part of it all as well. I sat next to her on a bench seat with our backs to the wall, we laughed the whole time and by the end of the meal we were holding hands. I drove her home and walked her to her door.

We were still holding hands as we turned to face each other.

- I think you might be clinically insane - She said with a smile - But I like it.

- Lunacy is infectious - I replied - You should be careful.

She laughed quietly as she looked at me. I looked into her eyes; they stared back up at me, reserved yet available. Her mouth was slightly parted with her lips curling in expectant amusement. As I stood there, I put my hand in her hair and I eased her closer to me. We kissed, gently, tenderly and warmly; there was no doubt, no hesitation. We both wanted this, we had a desire to connect as if it was already a part of our history that we were now experiencing for the first time. It felt instinctively right and we stayed by the front door for a while, looking into each other's eyes, touching each other's faces, enjoying each other's presence.

I did not want to leave, but I also did not want to stay over, not yet anyway, that would be for another night not too far away. I wanted to cherish the moment, allow the build up to happen, give ourselves time to imagine how it might be. We knew where this would go, but tonight was not the night for conclusions, tonight was the night of innocence.

We kissed again before we said goodnight and she stepped inside; she watched me walk away as she stood in the doorway, her hand resting on the door handle. I drove home with a smile on my face and a thrill in my body, looking forward to our next liaison, which we arranged for two days later, the Thursday; I would be in the studio recording a song the following evening and so Thursday was the next available time that we could meet.

As it happened, I had to be in Beverly Hills during the day on Wednesday, so I called Jemma at work before I left my house. I could not wait to see her again.

- Hey, I know we are meant to be seeing each other tomorrow, but I have to come into your area today, I was wondering; do you get a lunch break?

I heard her giggle at the end of the line, and then, as quick as a flash, she replied

- Yes, I do. It's union rules, you know.

There was a smile in her voice.

- Okay, I'll be a little more direct - I said with a laugh - Can I come and take you for lunch?

- Yes you can, I'd like that - She said.

- How's one o'clock?

- Perfect.

How Angels Die - A Confession

I ran a few errands, then drove into Beverly Hills and parked near the entrance to her work. I walked into the Gallery through the double glass doors on the corner of the street. Photographs were everywhere; big and small, abstract and classic, they could all be seen through the enormous glass windows that faced Wilshire Boulevard and now I was in the midst of them.

Jemma was seated at her desk, which was alone, along the back wall facing the windows; she was working on her computer and did not see me walk in. I smiled at the receptionist and walked towards Jemma. I could sense the sales staff watching, wondering whether I was a potential mark, and so once I got to her desk I did not give her a kiss in case it was the wrong thing to do, even though I wanted to. She looked up from the screen and a smile spread across her face.

- Hi - She said - Can you give me just a minute?

- Of course - I replied.

I crossed the Gallery and looked at a photograph of a suspension bridge as Jemma finished what she was doing. A minute or so later, she joined me.

- A bridge - She said, sounding like a salesperson - Something that gets you across the water without getting your feet wet. It prevents drowning too. Quite useful sometimes.

I turned to her, amused by her commentary; she was smiling back at me.

- Actually, I do really like that photo - She said - It's a clever angle... Shall we go?

- Yep. After you - I said before whispering - Gorgeous.

She reacted with a smirk and then we walked through the showroom and out onto the sunny street to my 4-wheel drive Jeep Renegade. I opened the passenger door for her and closed it once she was seated. As I climbed in the driver's side I leaned over and kissed her on the cheek. She blushed.

- I was going to do it at your desk, but decided against it, for your sake - I said.

- Good call - She replied with a wry smile.

As I started the engine I reached my arm across the center console and took her hand in mine. She took my hand with both of hers and we made our way to the little French Bakery on Olympic Boulevard.

We sat outside taking in the warmth of the California sun. Neither of us ate much of the food on our plate, and the time we had together was over too soon. It was good to see her again; to be around her was relaxing, fun and easy. As I looked at her, as she spoke, I was drawn to her, taken in by her bright eyes and her smile, attracted to her energy, her warmth, her honesty.

- Do you like your job? - I asked.

- I do. But it's not exactly taxing. I get overpaid to answer the phone and type letters.

- How long have you been there?

- Since my second day here. The interview was tough though.

- Really?

- Yeah. I walked in, the boss looked me up and down, and he asked me if I could type. I said "Yes". He then asked when I could start, and I said, "Tomorrow, if you like", and that was it.

I began to laugh.

She continued

- So, I'm pretty sure I didn't get the job for my typing speed. What do you think?!

- Oh, I don't know - I replied - Perhaps he's very intuitive, a psychic maybe.

Los Angeles is full of people who exaggerate their credentials, who live a lie, and who blow everything out of proportion. To be with a girl, a woman, who told the truth was disarming and appealing. As we sat at lunch, on that sunny Wednesday afternoon, my world took a turn towards Jemma and all that she stood for. I was, I knew, with an equal, someone who could hold my attention, who would give fairly in every way, who was well-rounded and full of life. Slowly, my internal guard began to fall.

- And what about your family, why are you here? - I continued.

We had not covered these things when we went out to dinner, we were having too much fun joking around, enjoying the scene queens and the club kings, and I had not wanted to ask the predictable questions.

- Well, I moved here a couple of years ago with my then boyfriend, Rick, but within a month or two he decided he didn't like it and so he went back to Denver where he has a construction company. We had been together for five years and I think we just grew apart really. It was a last ditch attempt to make it work, but we are still friends. My Mom still lives out there, and my older sister Katie does too, they're very close. I live with Christina, my twin sister, who you will meet one day soon, I'm sure. Other than that, I don't really know why I'm here. I like the lifestyle and the weather, but I don't want to be an actress and I don't have any grand plans. What about you?

How Angels Die - A Confession

She had mentioned she lived with her sister, at dinner, but I had not gone into it with her, I did not realize she was a twin.

- My mum is a twin, and her twin has twins - I said - Funny that. Do you like being a twin?

- It's okay, I guess - She said - Not that I know anything different. But it was a little annoying when we used to have to always dress the same way and have the same exact haircuts. I think we ended up finding our individuality in our characters. Christina is a much stronger personality than I am. I tend to go with the flow and accept things as they are, she's a much harder person than me; she wants to be an actress, so she chose the more difficult path. I chose the safe route. The easy life... Why are you here?

I listened to her, almost mesmerized. She seemed to be able to succinctly describe a complicated situation, to make sense in a few words; she was not dramatic and she did not embellish the story in any way. My thoughts wandered until I realized she was waiting for me to answer her question which she had now asked twice. I was so intrigued by her answers to simple questions that I forgot to respond. I jolted myself out of my daydream and spoke.

- Well, apart from the music, I don't really know, I used to design clothes in London, and I do the odd voice over when they need me, but that's rare. I guess I'm open to just about anything; singing is my main thing though. I do whatever I want, whenever I want, most of the time.

- Lucky you - She replied.

- Clever me - I laughed - And I love the beach. It's amazing. Before I got here, I had never seen the sun, they don't have it in England, you know, although it might explain the odd claim of a UFO sighting on less cloudy days. Anyway, when I first got to LA, I asked someone, "Hey, what's that big bright ball in the sky?" and they told me it was called "the sun." I was completely dumbfounded and I fell in love with it straight away, it makes me so happy, especially when it's mixed with the sea and the sand.

She laughed and looked up at me as she finished her mouthful.

- You see - She said - Insane.

I was wearing a t-shirt that day and so more of my tattoos were showing. As we spoke I noticed Jemma looking at my arms and the tattoos that adorned them; they include many symbols and quotes. The patterns are designed to be more geometric than anything else, a crucifix, an Egyptian eye, triangular shapes mixed with words or tribal style figures, and then, the number 37 on my left bicep facing the front. Jemma looked at the number.

- Tell me; what does the 37 mean? - She asked.

How Angels Die - A Confession

I paused. For good reason. To anyone else I would have given my standard answer, I would say it was my lucky number and the conversation would move on. I have never been much in favor of explaining the meaning of my tattoos, I usually joke that I got them for one of two reasons - extreme vanity or severe self-hatred - and in all honesty I am not sure which is true, perhaps both. It just so happens that the 37 is a very meaningful tattoo to me, but the meaning is beyond most people's comprehension, an inconvenient reason that is hard to explain, even harder to understand.

I considered giving Jemma the standard lucky number response or some other vapid comment, but then I decided to tell her the truth; I wanted to see her reaction. I wanted to make sure that she really was as cool as I thought she was.

- It's the age I will be when I end my life - I said.

Jemma instantly burst into laughter, and then she stopped just as suddenly when she realized I was not joking.

- Really? - She questioned - Why?

Now for the reason, as inconclusive as it sounds.

- Because I figure by then I will have done everything I want to do, but I will not have deteriorated too much. Quit while you're ahead, I guess.

How Angels Die - A Confession

She looked at me; I could tell she was intrigued, and still a little unsure as to whether I was joking.

Since I had been a teenager I had decided that I did not ever want to be old. I had watched my brother slowly die and I had spent too much time in places that were full of fear, pain and sadness during his illness. For many of my most formative years I had been sent to boarding school where my life was not my own, and I did not really fit in anyway. I had looked at my sensible, proper family and seen what age brought to them - repetitive lives, poor health and discomfort; I looked at the world and I saw the same.

Everything I had seen and experienced was enough to make me want to die young, to be in control of my health and my death, to know my own timeline, to give myself a goal, to have some semblance of control in a world that seemed to me to be so unfair and unrelenting.

I am very aware that this last sentence must seem overly dramatic and a little off beat to most people. I have no doubt that my somewhat odd outlook on life and death must come as a slight shock, but I assure you that I am not a crack pot, I just try to view life for what it really is, not what I wish it was, and I enjoy taking the path that nobody mapped out for me. I wake up every morning with a smile on my face; and I often remind myself "I am happy, I am healthy, I am wealthy in abundance." However, this basic inner happiness does not stop me from seeing the reality all around me, which led me to having a 37 tattoo on my left bicep, facing forward in full view of the person I am talking to, who at this moment happened to be Jemma; sweet, light-hearted Jemma.

As I spoke, these same thoughts of why I had the 37 tattoo came into my mind, they were highlighted by the look on Jemma's face.

- Are you serious? - She quizzed.

- Yep - I said, nonchalantly - But don't worry about it, it's not something I worry about too much.

I cracked a smile to dissipate the comment I had made.

- I'm sure you don't. But it is a little worrying - She continued - How long have you felt like this?

- Since I was young - I quipped - I always thought thirty-seven was a turning point in life, the age where you are old enough to have experienced life and young enough to still enjoy it. My great aunt once said, "Old age has nothing to commend it, dear." I knew she was right and so I decided I would never get old. And anyway, none of us, none of this matters in the long run.

- But thirty-seven seems a bit young - She stated.

How Angels Die - A Confession

- Not when you're nineteen - I replied - It seems like a lifetime away, plenty of time to do what you want.

- So what started this... this brilliant plan? - She asked.

Again, I paused. Was I revealing too much too soon? Would she ever want to see me again after this? I decided that I may as well find out sooner rather than later.

- My brother died when I was fifteen from a terrible wasting disease that took years to destroy him. Initially I thought I would become a priest to right the wrong of his death, I thought that by turning to God I could make the world a better place, but then, once I aged a little the pendulum flipped to the other side and I decided that I couldn't support a God who would do that to my brother, my mother, my father or me - so I discarded the idea of God, of an afterlife, of there being any point to any of this. I decided that all the worrying and suffering was a big fat waste of time, because nothing matters in the end anyway - and since then my life has been a lot easier, and I'm much more relaxed.

She watched me; half concerned, half amused, completely confused, totally intrigued.

- You are the most interesting person I have ever met - She said, very slowly - You appear to be highly intelligent, but...

How Angels Die - A Confession

I interrupted her.

- I might be so sane that I'm crazy?

She smiled, then she nodded, and then she looked down at the table.

- I better get back to work - She said.

I wanted to talk to her more, to explain my life, to tell her about my brother, my parents, my family, my school life, but I knew that now was not the time; I just had to hope and trust that she would still want to see me, to hang out with me despite my views, opinions and peculiar desires.

I reluctantly took her back to work after our lunch. I opened the door of the car for her and held her hand as she stepped out. We kissed lightly and then I watched her walk back into the Gallery.

She had beautiful, shiny, dark long hair, full of bounce. Her dress sense was simple, elegant and interesting; she wore jewelry that complimented her clothing and shoes that lengthened her legs, giving her body a distinctively feminine sway as she walked. Another smile spread across my face as I stored the image in my memory bank, to be recalled whenever she crossed my mind, which was already becoming a regular occurrence.

As I look back on it now, there was no particular moment when Jemma and I made the decision to become boyfriend and girlfriend; we just drifted into a pattern that was both constant and unpredictable.

Perhaps it was after that Thursday dinner when I stayed the night and we made love for the first time, in her bedroom, the street lights coming in through the white curtains giving the room an orange glow, her body a perfect fit for mine. She was petite, she was toned, she was warm and soft, and we connected instantly with a deep understanding, giving and receiving. We loved being in each other's company and consequently we ended up spending most of our spare time together.

She disarmed me with her honesty and her independence. She seemed perfectly happy to be alone yet she was very comfortable in social situations. She was an individual, and I admired that. It took no time at all for us to be planning our days with each other in mind.

How Angels Die - A Confession

On the weekends we spent in Hollywood, we would lie in bed making love, watching movies, ordering food and taking it slow. And then, on the Monday morning I would leave early to go to the gym so that she could get up and get ready for work.

Jemma took her time making sure she was as immaculately turned out as possible and I was aware that she liked to do it alone, so I left her to it; otherwise I would have stayed and watched her, handing her the hairdryer, passing her the hairbrush or mascara, like I did on the weekends when we went out for breakfast. She was my absolute sweetheart who I began to call "Angel", and by her twenty-seventh birthday, a month later, I had written her a poem and we were on the road to an easy love.

I was born and raised in the countryside just outside London, England. I was sent to boarding school at the age of seven and a half, and I moved to another boarding school at the age of thirteen, where I remained until I was nearly nineteen.

I remember thinking, in my teens, the school I was at, the people I was surrounded by, were not my kind of people at all. They were held down by tradition, in denial of the real world, unable to fully express themselves, staid and stoic, unimaginative and unoriginal, unadventurous and averse to change. I felt completely out of place, and perhaps to assert my sense of freedom and expression I started a rock band when I was seventeen, and began playing gigs at other schools, in the clubs of London or at other venues around Great Britain. I decided that I wanted to do music as a career; I wanted to sing, to be on stage, to perform.

When I finished school, I moved to London; my parents encouraged me to go to University, which I did, but I continued to pursue my music career playing in any place that would allow it, recording in studios or even bedrooms to get as much music down on tape as possible. I left University after the first year because I decided that Philosophy was a waste of time for my future and I was, in my view, just being taught to learn everything parrot-fashion; I felt as though my own critical faculty was being crushed by my 'miseducation'.

I took only a few vacations over the next few years as I was afraid that the ever elusive record deal may be just around the next corner and I did not want to be somewhere else just in case it decided to appear at the moment I was gone. I came close, but never signed the dotted line to fame and fortune despite signing all sorts of other contracts. I worked in nightclubs and stores and even began designing clothes, but in the end I decided England was not the place that would bring success, either emotionally or financially, and so I left at the age of twenty-nine and had been in Los Angeles, or rather, Laguna, for a year. I was still writing, recording and playing music, I had teamed up with a guitarist named Charlie and we played gigs all over LA, Hollywood and the surrounding cities.

My days in Laguna were my own to do as I wished. I had saved up and invested enough money to not have to work for a while and I had a simple lifestyle with few extravagancies but with everything I needed to fulfill my dream of living as if I was on vacation - this had been the main reason for me to move to the beach. Why work to go on vacation when I could live as if I was on vacation by cutting my expenses and moving to the sun? Once I met Jemma, I would drive up to Beverly Hills whenever I could to take her out for lunch.

In my spare time at home, I had written a book entitled 'Marriage & How To Avoid It' - it was a tongue in cheek look at the institution of marriage and the drama it creates in society. If I ever mentioned the title to people they would often laugh, and if I ever got into a discussion about my anti-marriage views I was always amused when divorcees were more argumentative than married couples. I was enjoying my life, I liked to juxtapose the positions of society as it always made for interesting conversation, and I intended to get my book published one day, although there was no sense of urgency on my part.

From the beginning, Jemma and I were affectionate; never once did we drive in the car without holding hands. We always, without fail, sat next to each other in restaurants - if there were only face to face tables available, then we would go somewhere else because sitting opposite each other felt like being in an interview, and holding hands across the table was awkward. We used to laugh about our little idiosyncrasies which were often compatible because we were interested in the same things.

I was interested in fashion, so I was more than willing to go shopping with her before or after we ate; at that time she had a serious shoe fetish and so I would have to make myself available to approve her next, slightly radical purchase from Diavolina on 3rd. If I had written a new song, I might sing it to her as we drove - she would be the first person to hear it and I valued her opinion more than any other. When her boss was out of town, we would, more often than not, use his office to fulfill our carnal desires before or after we had eaten; she was an open-minded, enthusiastic and talented lover - I looked forward to our lunch time liaisons, they were the brightest part of my day.

In the evenings during the work week, I would often stay with her in Hollywood, where we would go out to dinner, meet up with friends for drinks and visit the odd nightclub (which we would both want to escape from as soon as possible); or she might come down to Laguna so we could go to the movie house in the small town after eating in one of the myriad of restaurants. On the nights when we stayed in, we would attempt to cook an edible meal. If I had been particularly well behaved, I might even be treated to home-made brownies for dessert, which were my favorite because she always managed to make them stay soft in the middle.

- I know you think I'm a great cook because I can make brownies the way you like them - She said - But it's really because the oven is messed up and won't cook the middle properly.

It amused me when she spoke like this. So honest and humble, she would not even take credit for something as simple as a brownie.

We would often talk about and critique life in general, and more often than not we would discover how similar our views actually were, even if our delivery was a little different.

- Do you want to have kids? - I asked her one day over lunch.

- No. I don't think so. I mean, they're okay for an hour or so, but after that I have to run away - She replied - A little girl was in the Gallery today, actually, and she made me laugh. I was talking to her and she said, "Can I see that maZagine?" So I said, "Don't you mean maGazine?" And she said, "Yeah! MaZagine!" I can't stop laughing about it, she was adorable, but I was quite happy to let her go when the parents took her. Kids are such a handful.

How Angels Die - A Confession

From that day forth we always called magazines, 'maZagines'.

- And marriage? - I questioned.

- Not necessary - She continued - A nice idea that doesn't seem to work too well. I don't put too much thought into it, really. And I don't think I ever have, not even as a child, it was never something I focused on. I mean, other people's track records aren't too encouraging really, are they? I was never the little girl that wanted the fairy tale wedding.

- Me neither - I replied, smiling.

She laughed. Then she carried on with her thought.

- And to tell you the truth, my idea of hell is having to spend every day with one person. I just couldn't do it; I value my quiet time too much. I love being alone, being able to gather my thoughts without having someone else walk in the room and disturb me. I don't think I could ever live with anyone again.

- Where did you come from? - I asked - I think you might be perfect. That's exactly how I feel. I really believe that space is the essence of a successful relationship. Without it you have complacency and suffocation.

And there we had it. We were on the same page of the same book when it came to relationships, and it had taken us less time than it took most people to say "I love you" to figure it out. She really was perfect for me.

Since I had left England I had really tried to work on myself, to work out what it was that worked for me, what I was looking for in life, what made sense to me; I tried to think outside the box both emotionally, physically and financially, to create opinions that I made up for myself, to discard what I had been taught in favor of what I knew to be true. It had been a process and it was still a work in progress for me, but I knew I was making headway and I relished the idea of being able to discuss these thoughts and ideas openly with someone who was as prepared to question the world as much as I was.

I had found most people resistant to the idea of change or to the possibility that there may be another way to look at life, Jemma was as open and interested as I was which made our time together all the more enjoyable and stimulating; we were mentally and physically compatible. And so, although we considered each other in our daily routines, we still made sure to have our individual time and our freedom, which was made easier because we lived quite far apart, yet we maintained contact throughout the day even if we did not see each other. She was usually the first person I spoke to in the morning, and always the last person I spoke with at night.

How Angels Die - A Confession

If she had spent most of the week in Hollywood, Jemma might call me on Friday afternoon, her voice alive and free.

- Hey, can we spend the weekend in Laguna? I want to see the dolphins and listen to the waves. It would be good to forget about the world, wouldn't it?

- Yes it would, Angel. I'll be here waiting for you.

She would escape from work a little early if possible and come down to my white walled, wooden floored beach house, where the windows and doors opened up directly onto the sand and the ocean air was refreshing for her after a week in the city heat. We would go ocean kayaking to see the dolphins close up, or we would simply relax, read and sleep in the cool ocean breeze.

Sometimes I would lie with my head on a pillow between her legs and she would sit up behind me gently massaging my face as I drifted off to sleep to the sound of the waves. At other times I would tickle her back for hours and hours before we even got out of bed.

We were spoilt for choice, but we never took it for granted and we never failed to remember how peaceful these times were; it was our first choice to live this way and we were happy.

How Angels Die - A Confession

Being with her was always a pleasure, and as afraid as I was of falling for her, because I valued my freedom with intense determination, whenever I looked at her I was certain that I did not want to be without her. She was a beautiful person, inside and out, she was always looking for the good in any given situation, and if it was anything other than that, she would invariably analyze it with humor and clarity. Her character, although quieter, suited mine perfectly, while physically she was outstanding both to look at and to touch.

And then came that moment, I remember it as if it was yesterday - we were in her apartment in Hollywood, it was a weekend, in the late morning as the day began to heat up. We were lying next to each other on the bed deciding whether to go out for breakfast or to stay where we were for a little while longer when the phone rang on the opposite bedside table. I will never forget watching her crawl on all fours across the white sheets in her underwear to answer; she was in a midnight blue lace bra and panties, she was tanned, her stomach was tight and flat, the rest of her body was curvaceous and womanly. She glanced across at me with a wry smile and our eyes met; my eyes gave away how much I was enjoying the vision, her movement was so graceful, her manner so lovely. I was mesmerized by her, by her grace, her smooth energy, her demeanor, the way she answered the phone. I wanted time to stop, I wanted to reach out and touch her but I did not want to shift the moment from the idyllic image that it held - and in that instant I felt sure that this was 'it', she was 'it', being with her was 'it' for me - that was the moment I gave up fighting my insecurities and allowed myself to love her without fear. I knew she deserved it and I wanted to welcome her into my heart. I also knew that she would protect my heart with hers, she would love me fully, and I, in turn, would give her the best of me.

I never told her about that moment, the moment I fell in love with her completely. I do not know why, but I wish I had, just so she would have known how strong it was for me, how fulfilling it felt to be completely certain that she was what I wanted, in every way.

After this epiphany, and after we had been together for a few more months, I suggested that she come sky-diving with me. I had been a couple of times before and I thought it would give her a thrill. As I mentioned it to her, I could see the hesitation creep across her face, she was contemplating the actual moment of being airborne, hurled from the plane, nothing but a cold wind rushing past her, helpless until that parachute would burst open and the loud velocity of gravity would turn into weightlessness and an eerie quiet; but her eyes slowly lit up and her mouth began to curl into a smile.

- You see. Here we go again with the insanity - She said - Sure. Let's do it.

- Really? - I questioned, hopefully.

- Of course - She said - I'll do it. Once.

I laughed in disbelief, but I knew she meant it. It was settled. There was no back and forth with Jemma, no overtly analytical questions, no panic stations, just a second or two of contemplation and then a decision. If she liked the idea then she might as well try it, she might as well enjoy it, she might as well be with me - and so, one Sunday morning a few weeks later we drove out to Perris, California, we took the one hour de-briefing course, hooked up to our professional 'buddies' and we jumped out of an airplane from thirteen thousand feet; me first, her second. At five thousand feet we pulled the rip-cords and floated for a few minutes before landing safely back on terra firma. She loved it. She was dizzy with excitement and she could not stop laughing about it. On our drive back home along the 60 freeway we saw a drive-thru Krispy Kreme on the opposite side of the road.

- Look! - She exclaimed - I've never seen one of those before!

- Do you want to stop? - I asked.

- Yes, yes, yes. Can we?

- Of course we can, Angel.

And so we double-backed on ourselves, we pulled up to the drive-through window and we celebrated our new adventure with a box of twelve assorted doughnuts, which we began to devour in the parking lot. As we licked our lips and smiled at each other she said

- I have an idea.

How Angels Die - A Confession

- You do?

- Yes. Let's make this an annual event.

I looked at her and I began to laugh.

- Okay - I replied - Deal.

It impressed me that one so delicate and so elegant would be 'up' for such an activity, but it was just another side of her that added to her qualities. She genuinely wanted to be adventurous and she lived with a clear sense of extracting the most out of everything, as would be displayed when we went away to Hawaii.

It was her boss's second wedding, we went to Maui for four days and in that time we saw the sunrise at the top of the volcano and rode bicycles all the way down. We went scuba-diving and then followed the dolphins in the boat. We flew in a helicopter over the waterfalls and beaches and then we drove around the island in a car. We hiked, we lay in the sun and we attended the wedding ceremony followed by a reception; we did not have one argument and we made love whenever we could. On the flight home, as she rested her head on my shoulder and slowly drifted off to sleep she said

- Baby, that was fun, but I think we might have overdone it a little... What do you think?

How Angels Die - A Confession

- A little? - I replied - I think we overdid it completely.

- We got sucked up in the excitement and now I'm so tired I can't even think straight... Do you mind if I sleep on your shoulder?

- I would love you to.

- I like it when we take it easy and let the day unfold naturally; all that running around makes it feel like a job - She said with a giggle.

- I'm with you on that - I replied - I am with you on that.

We drifted off to sleep, and once we had landed we went back to the beach and spent the next few days in Laguna; she would get up in the mornings as the sun was rising and I would make her a sweet, sugary coffee and a bagel with butter and jam on it while she took a shower and got ready for work. I would talk to her as she did her final bits and pieces before leaving, and then I would spend the day at home working on my music, writing some lyrics, re-arranging a chorus, walking on the beach, clearing my head; nothing too strenuous, but always something that made life a little better, a little more perfect. We would talk during the day, easy talk, catching up, telling funny stories; and then, after work she would come back to my place and we would walk on the beach arm in arm before having a quiet evening listening to the sound of the ocean, taking life slowly, relaxing together.

How Angels Die - A Confession

There were times when she would question me regarding my rather extreme views on life and death.

- So, really, you just want to die at thirty-seven, that's it? - She might say.

- Yes - I would reply - I know it sounds crazy to you, but to me it makes sense.

She would sit silently for a moment before asking more questions.

- And what about your mother? Or your friends?

- I can't live my life for them - I would reply, quick to answer - They'll cope, I suppose. We all do in the end.

- And how would you do it?

- Pills. I don't want it to be too dramatic; I would like to slip away quietly. No mess.

- Are you depressed?

- No. Not at all. My mum always used to say that I must be a happy little fellow because I sleep with a smile on my face.

- You do! That's true. So then, why?

- Just because - I would continue - I know I'm lucky, I'm healthy, I have a good life, but I don't want to live past my expiration date, I want to make sure I'm in control of my own demise.

- I still think that thirty-seven is a little too young - She might retort.

- It's old enough for me - I would say with a smile - And it's plenty of time to do whatever it is I might do. Plus I wouldn't have to live with the regret too long if I ever did anything to regret.

We would laugh for a moment.

- It's not very fair if you have kids, though.

- I agree - I replied - And that's why I wouldn't have kids. As much as I love kids, I like that other people have them, I get to enjoy them or destroy them and then I can give them back once the sugar rush takes a hold. Being the once-in-a-while uncle is perfect for me.

She would smile at my planned answers.

- Well, don't you have it all figured out?!

- Yes I do - I would reply - I heard a saying once, "Most people learn very little in life, some people learn from their mistakes, and a genius learns from the mistakes of others." I want to be a genius.

- And that's why you want to die young?

How Angels Die - A Confession

- Old age has nothing to commend it - I would say.

Jemma never judged me for my lunacy; she simply listened, absorbed and moved on. Perhaps this was why we worked. I could express myself and all my off the wall ideas and she could be objective and laugh at me with her smiling eyes.

A few months into our relationship, I turned up at her apartment and she said

- My boss needs a new car driven up to San Francisco for his dad. He asked me if we wanted to do it; he will pay for a hotel in the city and then we will drive his dad's old car back down. What do you think?

- Sounds good to me - I replied - If you want to do it, I do. It should be fun, right?

- I think so - She smiled - I'll tell him yes.

We left on the Friday morning and we drove up Pacific Coast Highway until we had to take the freeways into San Francisco. Actually, I drove most of the way, and Jemma, after a couple of hours, lay in the back seat trying to sleep, while I kept interrupting her.

- Oh my God, you have to see this! - I would exclaim - It's so cool... Look at the ocean crashing against the sheer cliff below us!

How Angels Die - A Confession

Jemma would, initially, sit up to look and then lay back down, but after a while she just lay there, sleeping, or at least pretending to sleep while I drove along talking to myself, and her.

- Comfortable back there, are you, dear? Anything I can get for you? A duvet? A pillow? Cuddly toy?

I thought I was being quite amusing and I could see her suppressing her smiles when I turned around to look at her. But, after a while she basically ignored me, or pretended to be snoring to get her message across, which was probably wise.

When I was a child, my mother's recurring theme with my friends was, "Don't encourage him." I was relentless once I got hold of something that amused me, but Jemma had learned the lesson without ever having met my mother - although she would soon and they would become quite close over the years, the three of us spending birthdays and holidays together whenever my mother came to visit, which we all enjoyed because, luckily for me (and Jemma), my mother is amazingly relaxed and easy company.

When we finally arrived in San Francisco, we could not find the house we needed to deliver the new car to and so I asked Jemma to drive the last part of the journey as I was tired and irritable now that we were lost. As soon as Jemma got behind the wheel, she pulled out and nearly caused an accident - I immediately offered to drive again as I figured that it was better to be safe than sorry, but she insisted she was okay and finally we found our destination.

Once we had swopped over the cars, we drove to the Huntington Hotel on Nob Hill and had a fantastic weekend lying in bed until late in the morning, ordering room service, wandering around the streets of San Francisco, taking the small ferry to Sausalito, riding the trams and enjoying the city vibe, making sure to take lots of time over meals and regular breaks for coffees, smoothies or sodas. On the Sunday afternoon we drove back down to Los Angeles and collapsed into bed early on Monday morning before delivering the old car to her boss once he was at work. It was our first big road trip together and we had had a great time. We did not know it then, but it was in fact to be our only road trip together.

As the months went by, we grew to totally understand and respect each other for our beliefs and our love. I was still relatively new to Los Angeles life, I was trying to advance my music career and my hours were, more often than not, quite erratic. Jemma always welcomed me into her arms at the end of the night; she would leave the keys to her apartment under the mat and I would crawl into her bed even if she was already asleep. I was keen to sleep next to her so that I could wake in the morning and kiss her on the lips when I left.

In the early light of day she was very lethargic and dreamy so I would be very quiet as I left the room, but

How Angels Die - A Confession

I would always make a point of kissing her goodbye; she would be wrapped up warm under the covers with just her head on the pillow exposed to the chill morning air. As I leaned down to kiss her, she instinctively knew where I was and would turn her head to face me so that I could kiss her on the lips, but she was so sleepy that she did not actually open her eyes or move her lips at all, she simply allowed me to kiss them. I would always hold the kiss for a few seconds, and then, as I pulled away, her head would turn back to the pillow so she could resume her soft and warm morning slumber; it was one of the most endearing parts of my day for a full seven years, it was so unique, the way she was so aware and confident of my love that she knew where I was when I leaned down to kiss her, and she was so full of love that she lifted her head up just a little even though she was too peaceful to open her eyes. When I think about it now, my heart aches to experience it just one more time, to feel that love for just one more moment.

Before I walked out of the apartment on those mornings, I would always write her a little love note on a piece of white paper and would leave it on her bedside table. Sometimes I would hide another one in a drawer or in her purse so she would find it later in the day - a little surprise. I liked expressing my feelings, because I knew that she genuinely enjoyed the messages I left for her and it was important for me to know that she knew the way I felt about her. Over time, she bought little books with blank, colored pages so I could write the notes in them and she could have all my words of love and affection in one place. She would leave the book out each night in the same place so I did not have to go searching for a piece of paper in the dim morning light.

There was not a night I spent with her that I did not write her a note, and in all of the years we were together; she never forgot to leave the book out for me or to thank me during the day for my "sweet words." I still have every one of those notes. She kept them all. Loose pieces of paper, napkins, the post-its and booklets; every single one reminds me of how lucky we were to have had such a clear and demonstrative love.

We did not tell each other that we loved each other too often, Jemma always used to say that the more we said it the less it meant. I was not sure that she was right but I tried to make sure I only said it when it was appropriate for her, even if I wanted to say it more. I admired her strength of character and her ability to allow me my freedom. In return, I kept the "I love you's" to a minimum and I made sure to give her space when she needed it.

We loved freely and happily and willingly without saying it too much. I suppose, in the end, we did not really need to, we were very open with our affection and we never questioned our dedication to the other's well-being.

How Angels Die - A Confession

Much of what I felt for Jemma was never said, it was simply expressed by my actions, by our laughter, by the warmth we felt in one another's company.

7

Jemma was a very pragmatic person, which I admired. She understood me completely, encouraged me totally and loved me unconditionally.

The first few months were easy and fun. We meandered within each other's lives and we managed to still keep it fresh despite near constant contact. We just worked perfectly without it being perfect, because nothing is perfect and we both knew it without being bothered by it. We enjoyed being with each other and that was all that mattered. I loved the way she moved, the way she carried herself, the way she dressed, the words she used, the thoughts she expressed. Jemma was self-assured, yet meek and polite, her touch was gentle and there was a tenderness in her manner; she was delicate but not fragile; opinionated yet wise and diplomatic.

By nature, Jemma and I had similar dispositions towards the outside world - as much as we could socialize when the occasion arose, we were both just as happy, if not more than happy, to be alone, or with one another, nestling down to an evening at home.

How Angels Die - A Confession

On one particular winter evening, we had come back to her apartment from a quick shopping trip and we were easing ourselves into a quiet night in; Jemma had changed into sweatpants and a tank top, I was on the sofa in jeans and sneakers. I had just given her a necklace - it was a silver love heart on a chain with an 'I' engraved on one side and a dot on the other.

We had a signal for when we were too far apart to talk - we drew an 'I' in the air, then a love heart and then we pointed at each other.

When I left her a note, I often ended it with

I ♥ ·

which was derived from our visual signal of love - this was what the necklace signified.

- Thank you - She said - I love it so much. You are so clever... Thank you.

I put it on her neck and she touched it gently, smiling to herself.

A little later, as she went into the kitchen to see what was in the fridge, I noticed that she held onto the door frame to balance herself.

- Are you okay, Angel?

- Yes, just my balance is a little off today.

How Angels Die - A Confession

- What do you mean? Is that normal?

- For me, yes - She replied.

I was confused. How could that be normal? Why had I even phrased it that way? And her reply - what did that mean? I remained on the sofa and waited for her to return; I was a little concerned.

When she came back into the room, I asked her what she had meant by her comment; she was hesitant in her reply, but after a few moments she stated, quietly

- I have Multiple Sclerosis.

Her eyes were cast downwards, she went silent but I had a sense that she wanted to say more.

- Go on - I said softly.

- Well, a few months ago I was diagnosed with a mild form of MS, it was just before I met you. I had woken up one day, a few weeks before and the whole right side of my body was completely numb. I couldn't feel a thing. As the morning passed, the numbness disappeared and I was back to normal. Then a few weeks later I woke up and I couldn't see, I was completely blind - there was nothing but blackness. And again, as the morning went by, it got better, my sight returned and I could see clearly again; but that time really worried me and so I went to the doctor to have some tests, all sorts of tests, and they finally told me what it was. And there we have it. I'm twenty-seven years old and I have MS.

I sat there in stunned silence. She had spoken as if she was talking about the sales charts at work, no words were emphasized, no meaning was attached to any one phrase in particular, she was simply telling me the facts, but something in her voice alerted me to how serious this was, how shattering this diagnosis must have been for her.

I knew very little about MS; my uncle had nearly married a woman who suffered from it, and she was now in a wheelchair, only able to drive a car that had been specially adapted for manual use, no foot pedals at all, disabled for life with no hope of a reprieve.

I remained silent but I reached my hand over and took Jemma's hand in mine. I looked into her eyes. She looked back down at the floor. We must have sat there for a full minute without saying anything. I was at a total loss for words, I was aware that this was better than saying the wrong thing. But I could not just sit there, defeated by half the story, I wanted to know more, I wanted to help. If I could.

- So, what does that mean? - I asked quietly.

- I don't know - She said without looking up.

- Is there anything we can do?

How Angels Die - A Confession

- Well, I take medication for it, and so far it seems to work. Once in a while I have an off day, but it's not so bad.

She was being very brave about it, I could tell, and she seemed to be so accepting of the challenge and the uncertainty. I tried to imagine what it must be like to wake up every morning not knowing whether you are going to be able to stand up with ease, or whether you are going to open your eyes and see nothing, nothing but darkness.

- And how do you feel about it?

She looked at me, raising her eyes slowly, tears welling up as she struggled to make light of such a devastating revelation. I felt her pain, deep in my soul, it ricocheted through my body.

- Scared.

As she said it, my eyes welled up with tears too. I was heartbroken for her that she had to deal with this fear on a daily basis, and I was amazed that she dealt with it so gallantly, so silently. I had no clue until that evening, but now that I had discovered it, I only loved her more.

- Angel, I love you. I know you don't like me to say it too much, but I just want you to know that. And I also want you to know that... whatever I can do, you only have to ask.

How Angels Die - A Confession

The tears that had surfaced in her eyes now broke loose and streamed down her cheeks. I leaned forward and I gently pulled her towards me, into my arms, her forehead fell against my chest, I held her there; she sobbed quietly as I kissed the top of her head and stroked her hair. My legs were numb from the emotion I felt for her, an emotion I find hard to explain even now, it was so physical, so all-encompassing, so powerful, so totally confusing. The moments drifted helplessly.

- It doesn't scare you away? - She eventually said - I was so afraid to tell you.

My heart ached as she said these words, my stomach tightened, my throat went dry.

- No. It doesn't scare me. I'm here for you and I'm staying here with you. You are My Angel and we will do whatever we can to make this as easy as possible for you.

As I spoke, she raised her head and she kissed my cheek. She held me tightly, I felt her warmth against me, I felt her tears on my face, and I knew then, at that moment, we would fight this battle together. Jemma had found, in me, a support system that she could rely on, someone who would help her when she needed it, who would do her running around if she wanted me to, who would give her space when required, who would love her always.

How Angels Die - A Confession

I thought about how complicated it must have been for her to have found a boyfriend with whom she had so much fun, whom she loved dearly and who loved her in return, yet she had this 'secret' - this fearful, intangible part of her that might alter the whole situation, might scare me away.

As I put myself in her place, my admiration for her grew and my desire to be with her magnified. She was a person to be loved, someone whom I felt I could entrust with my love, and in return I wanted to be there for her in any way that I could.

We did not need to say anything more, we sat quietly as the evening turned into night, attached to each other on the sofa, linked with a common goal and a common enemy, finding comfort in our togetherness.

Despite Jemma's monumental revelation and the knowledge that she was fighting an erratic and difficult disease, she made it very clear that she did not want a fuss made over her.

- I really don't want to talk about it too much - She stated - It's here, it's a part of my life and it's something I will deal with. Talking about it won't change anything, worrying about it will only make it worse, so, if you don't mind, I would like to just pretend it doesn't exist. Is that okay?

- Yes, Angel - I replied - Whatever you want.

We ignored the cloud as best we could and enjoyed the silver lining. We continued to be as active as before, spending our time together, going to dinner, watching movies, relaxing at the beach. It was not until a few weeks later that anything truly frightening happened when I was with her.

We had gone to The Beverly Center in Los Angeles to see a movie and as we walked through the parking lot on our way out, she fell to the ground. It was not a fall that one would count as standard, it was not a stumble and then a fall, it was a sudden collapse, and the landing was hard; one moment she was up, the next second she was on her knees.

I could see that she was in pain and embarrassed. I saw the tears instantly swell in her eyes, my heart jolted with pain, my stomach tensed and my body shook with anguish. I wanted to hold her close, make sure that she knew she was loved and adored. I wanted to take away her pain. I wished time would stop still, that the people around us would disappear, that I could envelop her in my arms and protect her, care for her, carry her to safety - but that was not what she would want; I knew that.

Instead of my natural urge to over-react, instead of being overly-protective, I behaved as I knew she would want me to, I simply leaned down towards her, took her by the arm as gently as possible and helped her up to her feet. I made no comment as we walked carefully and slowly towards the car with her using me as a support while her legs were too confused to carry her. I then put one arm behind her back and my other arm under her knees as I lifted her gently into the car; once she was settled in the passenger seat I gave her a soft kiss on the cheek, took her hand in mine and squeezed it before closing the door.

We drove home in near silence, holding hands, eyes on the road; we deliberately avoided eye contact.

How Angels Die - A Confession

Every so often I would glance over at her, hoping to be able to reassure her that it would all be okay, but she was staring straight ahead. It seemed as though she was re-living the moment, incredulous that it had happened, aware that it was a reality, searching for an answer that she could not find. I made no effort to break her trance, I just let her mind try to unscramble what had just happened and allowed her the time to gather her thoughts and process the information. I was aware that she did not want to be disturbed, she did not want to hear false words of positivity or standard phrases designed to avoid the truth. I left her to her inner contemplation and turned back to watch the road ahead.

When we got to her building I helped her out of the car and to the door of her apartment; when she had unlocked the door and we were inside she went straight to the bathroom to clean up, with her hand sliding along the wall for support, the rest of her body rigid as she retained her composure. I knew better than to fuss over her as she walked, but I followed her in to help, and as she sat on the edge of the bathtub she lifted her trouser legs and showed me her knees; they were slightly cut and severely bruised.

- Attractive, right? - She said with a half smile.

I got down on my haunches in front of her. I bent forward and carefully kissed the bruises. Then I looked up at her and smiled back. She kissed me on the lips, she held my face in her hands and we rested our foreheads together as I interlocked my arms softly around her legs. There was no use saying anything, it would not help and it would not change anything anyway. All she wanted was to know that I was there, physically there, a presence that understood, a companion who did not question her.

We were silent, we just held each other.

- There's some hydrogen peroxide in the cupboard over there, and some cotton wool - She said after a little while.

Once she had changed out of her clothes and we had tended to the damage, I sat her on the sofa and brought her a can of Diet Coke with a straw - a little treat for My Brave Little Girl, a silent medal of solidarity. Jemma accepted it with a smile and a giggle - she liked to drink with a straw, even hot tea and coffee, she said it kept her teeth white, which always made me laugh; hence her amusement when I played into her little nuance.

In a strange way, this incident, as horrible and shocking as it was, made things easier; I felt better knowing what she was dealing with, although I wished it would just go away so she never had to worry about it. Now, in some odd twist, we were linked with a common realization, clear about the reality of her situation, the suddenness with which a day could change from great to awful.

I think it was also a weight off her mind, I had seen and dealt with, first hand, everything that she needed me to know, and she was now safe in the knowledge that we could handle these episodes quickly and quietly. I instinctively knew that she did not want to discuss it - she wanted to deal with the results not the details, and I was there to assist in that goal.

Of the two of us, I was far more inclined to talk about it and be open with the whole situation. She preferred to let it be, as if not talking about it meant it did not really exist, which somehow I understood. Jemma was not one to dwell on the difficult parts of life, she saw the good side of most things, but on another level it was a little frustrating for me.

I was of the mind that discussing the issues might help us find a solution, or at least get everything 'out in the open', and despite feeling that I was doing the right thing for her peace of mind, there was always an element of doubt that I might not get every aspect of her care the way she wanted if she did not make it clear to me. However, I respected her decision to leave the subject alone unless she expressly brought it up, and consequently the silence prevailed and we did all we could to carry on as normal whenever she fell.

As the months turned into a year our life together flowed as if nothing was too much to handle. Our sex life was not as yet hindered by the MS. Only rarely did Jemma feel unwell, and on those occasions I would ask her what she wanted to make her feel better so that I could get it for her - it might be a Diet Coke, a Snapple or a Vanilla Iced Latte from The Coffee Bean & Tea Leaf - her wish was my command in these instances. The least I could do was bring her a treat and every time I did I was greeted with words of delight and thanks, as if she had never had a sweet drink in her life.

This was another of her attributes, her ability to make even the most simple pleasures seem special; and now, when I think back on all the presents she ever gave me, they were always cleverly thought out and beautifully packaged. She seemed to have a sixth sense with the gifts she chose, the wrapping she constructed, even the cards and words that accompanied them, everything was always just what I wanted and I always felt spoilt by the time I had finished opening all of the special and unique items.

How Angels Die - A Confession

In turn, she was always excited to receive gifts from me and she showed her gratitude in the most natural and childlike way, she was a gracious and joyful recipient and I would inevitably receive a Thank You card in the mail a few days later that made my efforts more than worthwhile.

As the years passed, we became expert gift givers with each other and we rarely needed any excuse to be either the giver or the receiver of a CD, a pen, a book, a box of mints, a sweet drink or some candy, whatever might catch our eye and be something that showed we were thinking of each other even when we were apart for only a few hours.

The love we developed was, I suppose, quite insular. We would go out and meet friends occasionally, have dinner with people that came in from out of town, or meet up with other couples if we were asked, but we rarely instigated these situations and although we were not exactly anti-social, neither of us felt the need to put our love on parade.

Our strength was in our unity as individuals; it was a quiet, private love that was strongest when we were alone which was how we kept it most of the time. At other times, when we had to socialize, and one of us did not feel like being a part of a group, we might go out separately and see our own friends without having to be a couple.

How Angels Die - A Confession

This solitude we enjoyed and reveled in was demonstrated best when, one weekend, we were driving through Beverly Hills and we pulled up at a traffic light next to my close friend, Michael, who I had been to the Alanis Morrisette concert with when I first met Jemma. I noticed him as he noticed us; he waved knowingly at Jemma who was totally confused by this overly familiar 'stranger'. She looked at me and saw me smiling at her and laughing with Michael, and so we pulled off to the side of the road to chat.

He jumped down from his big Ford Bronco and came over to the passenger window.

- Hello, Jemma - He said.

Jemma looked even more confused, and a little concerned; I was silent, watching her demeanor with amusement.

- I'm Michael - He continued.

Jemma burst into laughter.

- He talks about you all the time - Michael went on - But I was beginning to think he was lying about having a girlfriend because we've never met!

We all laughed, I put my arm around Jemma's shoulder and then she popped up with

How Angels Die - A Confession

- I seriously began to think that you were his imaginary friend, Michael, who he invented to sound popular. It's so good to meet you, and to know that he does have a real friend.

It was an odd scenario, Jemma and I had been together for over a year at this stage, and she had never met one of my closest friends. We chatted for a while by the side of the road, before going for a coffee in a little patisserie. Jemma and Michael got along very well, luckily for me. Afterward, we would make plans to meet once in a while, but only if Michael organized it.

My mother would come to visit about twice a year from England. She would stay with me in Laguna and if she was with me for a two week period then Jemma and I might take her to dinner in Los Angeles, or we might go to see a movie together.

Jemma was completely at ease in these situations and over the years the three of us spent many days and evenings together both in Laguna and in Hollywood. My mum adored Jemma; she thought the world of her.

- She is just such a sweetie - My mother said, when they had first met - Her sense of style is so elegant and she has the most wonderful giggle, she is completely endearing. I am so happy for you, darling. She is a lovely, lovely girl.

How Angels Die - A Confession

Jemma always used to laugh at my mother's very strong English accent and found the use of the word 'darling' particularly comical. When the three of us were together, Jemma spent most of the time amused by my mother and I going back and forth over my childhood antics and laughing at my accent as it became more and more English with each passing sentence.

Jemma and I never traveled to England together, and despite never having seen my mother's house, she instinctively knew what my mother would like when she bought her a gift. Whether it was a candle holder or a soap, she would always choose something that suited my mother 'to a T' (as they say). To this day, my mother always talks about Jemma's brilliant gifts that are dotted throughout her London home; reminders of happy times.

I, on the other hand, did not meet her mother or the rest of her family, other than Christina, her twin, for many more years. Jemma very much lived in her own way, away from Denver and her old life. She would occasionally make a flight back to see them over Thanksgiving, but only if Christina went too.

As far as I could work out, Jemma found her family a little 'small town', and although she loved her aunt who lived in Boston, with whom she would speak quite regularly, she only spoke to her mother weekly and it always seemed to be a duty not a pleasure.

Her mother would sometimes send gifts to the twins and on almost every occasion this happened Jemma would hold up the items that she pulled from the box and say, with a smirk

- And why would she think I would want this?

She did not say it in a malicious way, it was almost an incredulous comment filled with amusement as to why her mother wasted her time and money sending gifts that would serve no purpose other than to take up space. I think Jemma appreciated the gesture on some level, but it was a gesture that she did not really crave or need. The relationship she and Christina had with their mother was at best strained and at worst non-existent - but it was not something that either of them dwelt on; it was just as it was.

Other than these relationships and the friends that would come and go in our lives, Jemma and I had little desire to be around other people. We would plan our time together, and if we felt like seeing friends, then we would invariably 'get it out of the way' on our own. We might meet up later when the night was over or we would see each other the next night. The inter-mingling that so often occurs between couples and their friends was not something that either of us were concerned with, and perhaps this distance and separation was a positive part of our relationship as it allowed us to maintain a feeling of individuality and kept us well-versed in the telling of anecdotes about people that we had either never met or only knew slightly.

Jemma's friendships were, in a sensible way, not that important to her. She had shopping partners, or friends she might meet for drinks, but she would invariably be with them for only a few hours at a time, and rather than build up a relationship that became co-dependent, she would keep an arm's length between them. She would make sure to always be a step away from any drama that may ensue, and if someone became over-bearing or needy, she would avoid them until the friendship evaporated.

- I just don't see why every friendship has to develop into something so serious - She said, once - Why can't people take it for what it is? I am not here to solve your problems or be involved in your problems, I just like hanging out with you. Shouldn't that be enough? It always seems to turn into this whole big thing that gets blown out of all proportion. That's why I'm so scared to make new friends. I don't want them knowing everything about me.

And another time she spoke about her colleagues at work.

- They all want to know too much. They ask me how my weekend was and I always give them some vague answer to get them to leave me alone, but that's not good enough gossip and so I have to listen to them go on and on about their weekend, their kids, their garden. It's enough to make me scream.

We would talk often about human nature, family life, friendships, and we both felt the same about most of it.

- I'm happy that your kids are so amazing and unique, but I don't need to hear every word they uttered over a forty-eight hour period. Yes, your dog is cute, but could you please get it to stop sniffing my crotch. And as for your cat, it just peed on my sweater, I know you call it 'spraying', but I call it something else. We can be friends, of course, but please don't call me at 3AM and expect me to make you cups of tea because your boyfriend left you for the ninth time this month.

We were harsh, sometimes a little too harsh I am sure, but we tinted our disdain with amusement and we made sure to keep our anecdotes and criticisms to ourselves. We generally liked people and we genuinely enjoyed our friends' company, it was just that we enjoyed being together more and we saw no reason to deprive ourselves of something so good, especially when we found it so easy.

We were never short of things to talk about. Never did we have awkward silences or major disagreements. Jemma was amazingly up to date with the latest celebrity gossip, but she did not flaunt her "useless knowledge", she simply was able to answer any question I had about any person I might have a question about. She always knew which movies were coming out and had a wealth of information on the latest music, the funniest TV shows or the most outrageous fashion accessory. She became my 'up to the minute guide' on all things current, and yet I never saw her reading a gossip magazine or watching an entertainment program; it was always baffling to me how she attained and maintained her vast 'street' knowledge.

Peppered into these conversations were questions of mortality and humanity. Sometimes we would explore slightly uncomfortable subjects, but always with a light tone. I often spoke of my views in a way that may have seemed negative to others, although to me they were mere observations. She never made me feel defensive about the way I felt.

- It seems to me that we are just a bacteria - I would say - The human race has no respect for the environment that supports it. We are destroying our host as any good bacteria does; we have become vacuous, our lives filled with meaningless exploits like video games, televisions, movies, clothes, lazy pastimes that ignore all consequences.

Jemma would listen and sometimes interject; rarely did she disagree. I sometimes wonder if I spawned these ideas in her or if she already viewed the world this way.

How Angels Die - A Confession

- I know - She might say - It always makes me wonder what our purpose is when I see the traffic in LA and then I realize that every city in America has the same problems and every country in the world has millions of people sitting in their cars all day long; it makes me feel very insignificant.

- It's a sad truth - I would add - But the best thing for this planet would be the extermination of the human race.

She would laugh out loud at my unreasonable reasoning, but she would get my drift. We would often go over the state of the world, the point of life, the difference we did not make, and the stage at which it all might end.

- I heard that once we reach thirty our bodies are in decline anyway, slowly deteriorating with each passing day - She once commented uneasily - How depressing.

- Which only goes to prove my point that we should enjoy our lives, that there is no point getting stressed out over things we cannot control.

- Agreed - She would conclude.

And with our lives designed to travel along this simple and pleasurable path, it was easy for us to forget that Jemma harbored a disease that could instantly, inexplicably and literally bring her to her knees.

How Angels Die - A Confession

Perhaps this was why we maintained our air of semi-cynical yet amused disdain, perhaps this was why we kept ourselves to ourselves, perhaps we found strength in being a step removed from the social life of others, perhaps being insular allowed us to maintain some sort of control over what might be around the next turn in the road.

10

They say MS is often related to severe childhood trauma; if that is so, then Jemma most definitely experienced something that would account for her MS.

This is her story as told to me -

I was raised on a farm in Massachusetts with my father, mother, older sister, Katie, and my twin sister, Christina. I absolutely idolized my father, we both did, to the point where Christina and I would follow him around all day given the chance. I suppose he was our all-American hero and our rock, kind of like Superman. He was so strong and he was always working on stuff, so we would just sit and watch him. We probably annoyed him with all the questions we would ask but he didn't seem to mind and he would teach us things as the day went by; those are my strongest memories of him.

We used to have to go to church on Sundays with our dad's mother who lived across the fields in another farmhouse with aunt Laura. She was funny, our grandmother, very old fashioned. She called a sofa "a

Davenport" which we thought was very amusing. We used to dread Sundays and we would object to our mom about going to church because we found it so boring. When we complained that she never went to church so why should we, she always gave us the same answer

- I've paid my dues. You have to pay yours.

She was so irreligious in those days, like she was angry with God almost. She seemed to be kind of unhappy, as if she was depressed or something. She was originally from Denver, but after she married dad they lived in Massachusetts and she made it very clear she didn't like living there. I remember asking her why she agreed to live there if she hated it so much and she said

- Once you're married, you follow your husband no matter what.

Which I thought was very strange at the time, sort of like a martyr would say it. I liked her, generally, but as I got older I wondered why she had ever become a mother in the first place. She didn't seem to be very involved with us as far as I recall - it was mainly my dad who was at home. She kind of traveled or went away to visit people a lot, I think. I don't remember her being at the farm, she didn't really fit in there.

Christina and I were born on the exact same day as Katie, but three years later. I think she hated us from the moment we were born because we took away all the attention; two cute babies, adorable little twins everybody fawned over. She used to tell us that we were the worst birthday present she ever received! She was a bookworm, while Christina and I were far more lively. She hated the noise we made and the disruption we caused. Katie used to pretend we had done things wrong or she would break something and then blame us and we always got in trouble. When we got older we used to torment her mercilessly. She should have seen it coming; we were very cruel to her, like she had been to us.

Now we get along better. We live so far away from each other and we only meet up once a year or so. She's in Denver, near mom, and she has a daughter who's the apple of mom's eye. Consequently, Katie gets all the attention and time she needs, as well as a free babysitter. It's good in a way because it means that she takes all the attention away from us and we don't have to deal with mom so much.

One day, it was a school day, I think, when Christina and I were eleven years old. We were looking for dad but couldn't find him in the house or in the barn. I think we had found a note in the kitchen that had made no sense to us and so we were going to ask him about it. It said something like, "If I can't have both, I don't want either" and ended with the line:

Bang Bang, look who's dead
Johnstone shot himself in the head

How Angels Die - A Confession

Katie was with us while we were calling for him. We were getting further and further away from the main farm when we came across an old outhouse that was usually padlocked. It looked like the door was semi-open. Katie went in first but she instantly turned around. I distinctly remember her pushing Christina and I back out of the doorway telling us we couldn't go in; she had seen our dad, his head blown off by a shotgun. Later, she told us he was in a chair and the gun was still in his mouth. Anyway, we all ran back to the house as fast as we could to find mom but she wasn't around. We quickly ran to our grandmother's farmhouse across the fields.

There was a lot of commotion, people coming and going, the ambulance, the neighbors, strange visitors, and then over the next few days the preparations for the funeral. We were not really allowed to be involved in the grieving process; it was as if we were not allowed to know what had happened. We were completely excluded. A silent barrier separated us from the immediate family and from our dad's death. It was very confusing at the time and I remember feeling quite hurt by it.

Christina and I talked about it all the time during the immediate aftermath trying to figure out what had happened. Of course, neither of us knew anything because we had been told nothing. We were just little kids, and so we hid in our room, out of the way. We were sad beyond description and felt very lonely and scared. Christina was the only person I felt safe with at the time. I think it was the same for her with me.

After the funeral, mom acted as if nothing had happened and she sent us on a two week trip to Disneyland in Florida, like a vacation. We went with our grandmother. It's kind of a blank in my memory, but when we returned home we kept asking mom questions. She wouldn't answer them or she gave really vague responses. We were never allowed to see the suicide note again. I think she told us she had thrown it away, but we could sort of remember certain phrases he had used and so we asked her about those. She just pretended those things had not been in the note or gave us answers that made no sense. We knew she was lying, but she stuck to her guns and kept denying everything - almost as if she would believe it herself if she repeated the lie often enough - or it would then be the truth because she said it was. It was as though she was hiding something. I think she probably knew exactly why he killed himself but she didn't want to tell us and she never has.

I used to think about it all the time, but now it only comes up once in a while, and when it does I generally wonder why my dad did that. What was so awful that he felt he had to kill himself and why would he leave us without saying goodbye? I try to think back to see if I can remember him acting differently but I can't quite recall that time. I had an almost idyllic childhood up until then.

How Angels Die - A Confession

I think I'm angry with him too, for leaving us. Why would a father of three young girls just end his life like that, leaving us all alone without our daddy? He was everything to me, like a superhuman, and we just loved him so much. He left my mom without debt or financial hardship, but still, his actions were so incredibly selfish. It's hard for me to even like him anymore, in a way.

That was her story.

The first time I heard it I filled with sadness for her. I imagined these vulnerable twins, eleven years old, withdrawn and almost banished, in their bedroom, trying to understand what had happened to their daddy, what was happening to them, what was happening all around them.

Although she never said it outright, I am sure that she must have questioned how much their father actually loved them if he was prepared to leave them without even a goodbye, and therefore, she must have questioned her perception of him and her belief that he loved them as much as she had thought. He had basically ripped the foundation from beneath their tiny feet, broken their little hearts and left them in a tailspin that Jemma, for one, never fully recovered from. I think, for Jemma, the absence of any satisfactory answer or explanation about her father's end must have been a trauma that had no end itself. It must have effected her outlook on life in many ways.

How Angels Die - A Confession

It frustrated me that her mother had not been more forthcoming when her daughters had questioned her, but I would not attempt to judge the actions of a mother who loses her husband to suicide. No matter how prepared we are for death, we all react differently. When one is concerned for the welfare of three young children, the pressure of maintaining a normal existence must be frighteningly real and daunting. What I do know is that her behavior in the aftermath of the suicide was a point of contention and confusion for Jemma (and for Christina too) that was never concluded.

I also think this trauma was twofold for Jemma - her father's demise at his own hand compounded by her mother's lack of explanation to the point of denial. For a young girl, essentially in love with her daddy, this must have been incredibly difficult and frustrating to come to terms with.

I remember in the final days of Jemma's life, she was watching MTV as I completed some of the chores around the apartment, when the Kelly Clarkson video for the song 'Because Of You' came on. The song appears to blame her parents for her insecurities - half way through the song, Jemma burst into tears and said

- I don't like this song, it reminds me of my dad.

She leaned forward, picked up the controls and turned off the television.

How Angels Die - A Confession

To this day, I still hurt when I think of how useless I felt as I comforted those tears and that deep sadness. I sat with her on the sofa, spoke soft words of comfort and let her cry. I was well aware that her emotional pain went far beyond anything my hands or my words could support.

11

After we had been dating for a couple of years, Jemma was having a very difficult time living with Christina. They were not getting along too well and Christina was, I felt, behaving inappropriately towards Jemma - especially considering Jemma's condition, and knowing that stress was the last thing she needed when fighting the MS.

Christina had a wayward boyfriend, Paul, who was a journalist for some little known music magazines. Christina and Paul would come into the apartment late at night after having been to some gig somewhere; making unnecessary noise that woke Jemma and kept her awake. Christina would also 'borrow' Jemma's clothes without asking and then would either ruin them or keep them.

Jemma was quite upset by Christina's behavior, she felt unnerved by the intrusion into her sleep and into her room, but Jemma was such a meek and sweet person that she did not want a confrontation.

I, on the other hand, was at the end of my tether. Whenever I stayed over at the apartment, we would be woken by the noise that continued unabated even if we asked them to drop the volume. I was, I am sure, overly protective of Jemma, but I could no longer keep quiet.

- I don't understand why Christina can't be reasonable about the noise at night - I would say - And when she takes your clothes without asking, that's called stealing, Angel.

- I know - She would reply - but I can't stop her doing it because I'm at work, and I have asked her to just tell me so I know what she has, but she doesn't tell me. What else can I do?

Jemma did not want to cause a scene. She and Christina had always had a relationship where Christina was the more powerful twin; while Jemma was easy going, Christina was determined and headstrong, and she went after what she wanted whether it was right or wrong. It was the way it had always been, a dynamic that would not change now.

- Alright then - I said - I'll put a lock on your bedroom door so she can't get in when you're at work.

- It won't make any difference - Jemma replied - But if you want to, I won't stop you.

The day after I had attached the lock, Christina managed to break it and she had made no effort to hide the damage. She had rummaged through

Jemma's clothes and had taken tops, skirts and shoes.

Jemma and I came back to the apartment to find her bedroom door lock smashed and the handle on the floor, some of her clothes and shoes were scattered around the room. Jemma stood there in shock for a moment and then walked into Christina's bedroom. Christina was not home and so Jemma began to look through the room for the missing items. She found most of them hidden under the bed, on chairs or in drawers, randomly stuffed away, out of sight. She was angry. And so was I.

- Angel, this is outrageous.

- I know, but please don't say anything to her, she will only do something worse if you do, she always seems to take everything a step further and when she's cornered she lashes out. Please - Jemma begged me.

The twins had a history of ups and downs with their friendship. Jemma had told me that they had lived together once before and it had been a disaster, but when Christina had asked to try again, Jemma had acquiesced, which was why they were living together now. It was a decision she had not regretted at the beginning because Christina would spend most of her time at Paul's house, but now he had moved out of that house because he could not afford the rent, and he was basically living with Christina when he was not staying on a friend's couch.

Jemma liked Christina, and when they did not live together they got along very well, but the past few months had not seen Jemma's health get any better. In fact, walking around had oftentimes been quite difficult. The added stress of disturbed sleep, another occupant in the house, less privacy and a strained relationship with Christina all contributed to her feeling less than comfortable. I pushed for a conclusion to this issue.

- Okay. But if we have to keep quiet about this, I want you to move out, get away from her. I think she is stressing you to the limit and that's not good for your MS. I'll help you do it.

- We'll see - She replied, quietly.

I did not want to get caught in a battle between twins, but I could see the effect that the whole situation was having - Christina was only working once in a while, Paul was not making much money, and so they were on a different wavelength to Jemma who worked quite long hours and sometimes had to be available in the early evenings for Gallery events.

It was an unfortunate state of affairs, but after we discussed it further, Jemma agreed that it was not conducive to her maintaining her health and so, over the next few weeks, we looked for an apartment for her.

The efforts at searching for a new abode were, in my view, a little half-hearted, until one day Jemma opened the mailbox to find a court summons in her name, but she had no clue what it was for. Her instinct told her that this was Christina's doing.

Jemma's instinct was correct.

It transpired that Christina had been stopped by the police in her decrepit BMW without a driving license and without insurance despite being a nanny for a family whose children she drove to various locations; she had ended up in handcuffs face down on the tarmac, and in the heat of the moment she had given the officer in charge Jemma's name and social security number instead of her own, and had failed to inform Jemma. If Jemma did not turn up to the court date, which was less than a week away, she would have a warrant out for her arrest. When Jemma confronted Christina about the deceit, she heard

- I was going to tell you, I promise. I just forgot, I'm so sorry; I really was going to tell you.

- And when would you have told me, Christina? The court date is this Friday and this is the final reminder, which means you have been deliberately hiding this from me for over three months.

How Angels Die - A Confession

When Jemma told me about this I lost my patience and I told her that she had to step up her efforts to get away from Christina. Christina had obviously been hiding the paperwork and letters from Jemma to avoid having to tell the truth and she did not care what the consequences might be to Jemma's life, so long as she got away with it.

I was outraged and disgusted by Christina's behavior, and was more than willing to display my feelings to Jemma. At one point I even said

- You better keep me well away from her. I will probably do something we will both regret.

I remember Jemma's eyes looking at me with a mixture of disdain and irritation as these words fell from my lips; but I could not help myself, my protection mechanism towards Jemma was so strong that it was probably a good thing I warned her of my possible intentions. As it was, that look from Jemma was all I needed to know that it was time to back off a little and let her deal with it her way even if it was not what I would have her do.

Jemma went to the courthouse the day of the hearing and somehow extricated herself from the charge without implicating her twin.

- You are a better person than me, Angel. I would have sold her down the river for that one.

- I know. I know. But if I had, she would pay me back ten times worse. I know her, and I know how she works, it would just end up with her ruining my life some way or another.

Within a month Jemma had found a new place to live which was a block and a half away. The next weekend, when Christina was out of town, I moved Jemma's stuff from one apartment to the other.

I ended up carrying the bed base up the street and across Melrose because it was too big to fit in my SUV. As I came up the hill, lumbering slowly, slightly exhausted, arms stretched wide with a big black metal frame between them that was squashing my face Jemma burst into fits of hysterics. She could not stop laughing - she said it was the most ridiculous sight she had ever seen.

- But I love you so much for being so good to me. You are the best. Sorry I'm laughing, Monkey. You don't mind do you?

- No, of course not, My Angel. I'll forgive you, if you make me brownies.

When we had finally moved all her furniture in and she was settled, Jemma handed me a key to her new apartment.

How Angels Die - A Confession

- Just in case - She said with a smile - I promise I won't ask you to move in, it would be just as painful for me as it would for you!

- Thanks, Angel. You're too kind - I said jokingly, as the keys rested in my hand.

After having known each other for over two years, we were under no illusion as to how much we both valued our individual homes; even though we spent at least four nights a week together, we both felt that having our own space and the ability to use it was an important ingredient in the success of our relationship, so we were not about to change a system that worked so well.

- I feel so much better having my own place - She said a little later.

- Imagine the look on Christina's face when she sees that you are gone - I laughed.

- Oh God - She said - I feel bad again.

I did not miss a beat in reinforcing my point of view.

- She deserves it. And you know it.

Jemma was silent. As much as she hated to upset anyone, she knew that Christina had pushed her to this point of desertion and hiding.

Christina tried to contact Jemma to find out where she had moved, but Jemma avoided her for quite a while. It was not until a few years later that they reconciled fully. Christina was very forthright and apologetic about her behavior at the time. She had become embroiled in Paul's life and had felt a little lost, she realized that she had been less than helpful to Jemma and she seemed genuinely remorseful. Jemma was more than willing to forgive her twin sister and they ended up becoming quite close again.

I believe moving out was a good move for Jemma, it made Christina appreciate her twin and it allowed Jemma time to sleep, be alone and be at ease without the worry of someone invading her life and disrespecting her privacy.

- Well, at least I get to walk around naked now - She said.

- Can I have front row seats? - I asked - Or do I have to peep through the windows?

She laughed encouragingly.

- I'm so glad you did this, Angel. I think it's very important that you have space and time and no stress. We'll make sure you eat well too, but I do think you should reduce the amount of Diet Coke you're drinking; it's not good for your MS.

How Angels Die - A Confession

- I know. Please don't get on at me about this. I like Diet Coke; it keeps me awake and gives me energy.

- Angel, I had an eye operation that was the most painful thing I ever went through, worse than all of my tattoos put together, and I could have prevented it if I had just been sensible when I knew something was wrong. I'm only saying that prevention is better than cure, so if you can do things that are good for your body, instead of bad, then perhaps we can make things easier for you.

- But where do we draw the line, Baby? What does my life become? Do I only drink the milk of newborn fairies and only eat the apples that fell off the tree because otherwise it's murder? What do you want me to do?

I laughed. She was making it clear that I would not be able to change her mind, I knew it, but I said one final thing anyway, I couldn't help myself. I was deeply concerned that her diet was not adequate to help her fight her condition, and more than anything I wanted her to regain full health if it was at all possible. Although not terrible as yet, some things were definitely getting worse in terms of her walking and her balance and I felt that she could make small changes that might make a big difference.

- I just think that you need to be sensible. You have an illness that reacts to your diet on some level, so you should be a little more careful; drink less saccharin and eat more healthily.

- Alright. I'll try. But don't give me a hard time if I don't do what you think I should do. Please. Is that good enough?

- Yes, Angel. I'll pick my battles.

Most of the time, her joy for life and her wish to be happy would over-ride everything else. She would always downplay her illness; it was a genuine strength of character that allowed her to see the positive aspects of most things and to enjoy her time in the most genuine way. I sometimes felt I was more concerned about her MS than she was and I would be the one to make her take it easy even when she tried to get up and go.

A number of years before, I had had an operation for a detached retina which was the most stressful thing I had ever had to deal with. Being young and naïve, I had ignored the signs and the symptoms and had ended up having to have a long, painful and complicated surgery which could have been avoided had I been more vigilant. I made it my (sometimes slightly annoying) job to try to help Jemma prevent making the same mistake.

I know it was irritating for her when I became too conscientious, and so, often I would have to bite my tongue and allow her to live her life in the way she wanted. I think her attitude was more fatalistic than mine at the time and so she had decided to enjoy her days no matter what the consequences might be.

I would imagine that having MS made her realize how fragile every moment was and her behavior reflected a more 'laissez-faire' way of living than I was accustomed to, or might have hoped she would have, for her sake as much as mine.

I sometimes wondered if her father's death had something to do with it. Who was I to judge? I just had to remember that my role was to support Jemma, and nothing more.

During the first few months in her new place, we did what most couples would; we spent the majority of our spare time shopping for furniture and other items that would turn her apartment into a home.

Jemma did not want carpet so she replaced it with wall to wall bamboo matting. We found a lovely three seated antique-looking brown leather sofa and paired it with two old plantation chairs that had wooden frames and leather seats. Jemma went online and bought a coffee table and a side table that were very solid looking and were covered in leather with light stitching on the edges to contrast their bulkiness. We put tall plants in the corners of the sitting room and the bedroom to soften the atmosphere and dotted original handmade candle holders all over the house, with soft corner lamps for added ambiance. We dressed the bay windows with long, sheer, white curtains that let in as much light as possible whilst maintaining privacy from the street outside.

I had a wooden dining table made for her that matched the chairs she had found and I also had an eight foot by six foot wooden framed mirror made in time for Christmas that year. She bought a couple of Moroccan style bedside tables and a leather headed bed that was more comfortable than anything either of us had ever slept in. The TV armoire was a dome topped wooden cabinet that added softness to the solid furniture, yet suited it all perfectly.

The apartment was light and airy so we contrasted that element with dark or mid-colored woods and warm leather or suede. When she could not find cushions she liked for the sofa, we bought the fabric and the inners and then had my tailor sew them up with a contrast stitch; she loved these cushions, they were over-sized and soft and could be used as either a head rest if she was watching TV or as a lap pillow if she was reading a magazine or book.

By the time we had finished, I was an expert at do-it-yourself fixtures and furniture construction; on occasion I would get quite frustrated if something did not fit together properly or if the wall was too solid for the nails I had used. I was not afraid to vent my feelings. Jemma was very grateful for my help, but used to find my aggravation quite amusing and she began to call me her "Disgruntled Interior Designer" if my patience was wearing thin; it would always break the tension.

She used to assist as much as she could, but many of the jobs that needed to be done required strength and balance that sometimes were not available to her so I found it easier and quicker to do most of it myself. Once the decoration was complete we did not really continue adjusting or adding. We had set out with an idea and we had done what was needed.

- Thank you so much for all your help, Monkey. I know it was annoying sometimes, but I am so happy with it, I love it. I couldn't have done it without you. Really.

- It was my pleasure, Angel. I love your new little home too, and despite my sporadic impatience, it was worth every second, because we got to be together as we did it, right?

- Yes. Right, my Disgruntled Interior Designer. And you are invited to dinner whenever you so desire.

- Thanks, Angel. Let's hope you don't regret that invitation.

- Oh, I'm sure I will - She said - I'm sure I will... But I have no doubt that I'll need something done soon enough, so I better keep you well fed and happy.

Doing everything for the apartment had really highlighted Jemma's fragility. There had been times when she was not strong enough to help me carry things and she had to sit down while I did it alone. I surprised myself with my strength sometimes and I wondered whether I was able to do the work of two people because I did not want to make her feel any worse than she already did.

I felt privileged to be loved by her and I wanted to repay that love by making her life stress free as possible. The last thing she needed was to be made to feel any weaker than she already felt, and so, despite knowing the truth somewhere within us, we managed to shroud that truth by still achieving our goals in whichever way we could. If one of us succeeded, both of us rejoiced.

Despite this underlying worry about her health, we lived our lives with love and with an understanding full of mutual respect and enjoyment.

There was not a time when her condition became an excuse for her not to do something, and in this, she astounded me; even on days when I could feel that she was not at her best, she was not the one to cancel the plans or allow her condition to get the better of her.

Sometimes she might ask me to come to Hollywood so we could have dinner at her place rather than have her endure the rush hour drive along the 405 and Pacific Coast Highway into Laguna. She always delivered her request with a sweetness that put no pressure on me.

- Would you mind coming up to me tonight? Just if you want to...

She did not need to say anything more. I knew that she was not feeling good, and on top of that, I knew we would have a lovely evening of takeout food, treats and TV, accompanied by highly amusing conversation and a host of affection. So, the answer was always

- Not at all, Angel. I'll be with you as soon as I can.

As I put the key in the door to her apartment, I was always filled with a sense of excitement. There was something so nurturing about Jemma, and her welcome was, without fail, full of enthusiasm and happiness. She would invariably be lying on the sofa with a cushion behind her head and she would either be listening to music, watching TV or reading a book - whichever she was doing, she would break away from it and lift both her arms directly into the air as she smiled and said

- Hello, Monkey!

I would then close the door, put my overnight bag on the dining room chair and walk around the sofa to get on my knees and give her a big hug and some hello kisses. I would look into her pretty blue eyes that would smile back at me and I would put my hands in her thick hair that rested on the suede cushion as I allowed myself to study her randomly placed freckles, her immaculate eyebrows, the delicate bridge of her little button nose, her full lips and her perfect jawline.

I would marvel at how beautifully constructed her face was, it was the kind of structure that someone might pay to achieve, it was that faultless, and to top it all, her skin was as smooth and flawless as any I have ever seen. She truly was a pretty, pretty girl; she had a beauty that was enhanced by her inner goodness and radiance. As I allowed my eyes to follow every detail of her I would smile to myself in pure wonder.

- What's so funny, Monkey-chops?

- Nothing, Angel. You're just so pretty, it's ridiculous.

Then I would kiss her on the nose and lips and I would lie on the sofa next to her. We would be very tightly intertwined and we would stay holding onto each other for some time before one of us would interrupt the proceedings.

- Are you hungry?

- Yes.

- Grab the phone, let's get some food then.

12

Initially, the MS was limited to balance issues and some numbness on the odd occasion. Jemma took the prescribed medication on a daily basis - it became part of her routine in the morning.

Over time the MS took a slightly stronger hold of her system. Her legs gave way a little more regularly than usual and she would fall down in the middle of the sidewalk, or at work. She resisted being helped up - her pride was always dented by the offers and her clothes were often ripped by the fall - but she carried on gallantly and more often than not the only way I would know she had 'been in the wars' would be when I saw the bruises on her knees or a bloodstain on the floor. She always brushed off my concerned comments with a light-hearted quip and rarely wanted to give me any detailed explanations. Perhaps there was no explanation that would make either of us feel any better.

After about three years, her condition had worsened considerably and the frustration grew as the MS would not loosen its invisible grip on her body - it was not a constant issue, which made the problem far more difficult to deal with. There could be two full weeks where she seemed to be in perfect health and our hopes were raised that she might somehow have conquered the disease but then the following days might bring on a variety of symptoms that carried no logical pattern.

Yet, none of this appeared to matter with regard to our relationship and the way we were together. Jemma, being the sweetheart that she was, never once took it out on me, never became depressive and never wallowed in self-pity. I am not so sure I could have been quite so noble if confronted with the same obstacles on a random basis, but she was goodness personified in this respect and she only ever showed me happiness, smiles and love. To all intents and purposes, we were only mildly affected by her "once-in-a-while" illness. She was basically active and mobile at this stage and more often than not we would be able to do whatever we felt like doing together.

The fourth year was when her balance became a serious problem. MS was a daily concern and she would - on her "bad days" - slide her hand along the wall to remain upright because she could not trust her legs to hold her. Staircases were no longer a few steps; they became mountains that required deep concentration to negotiate.

In years five and six, these bad days became more and more frequent until everyday could be classified this way. To watch her struggle was heartbreaking, but struggle on she did despite the anguish she silently went through. Whenever I was with her I would hold her as firmly as I could without seeming to be too involved. As we approached a staircase I would walk slowly in front of her so she could hold my waist when ascending or rest her hand on my shoulder when descending.

In general, she would no longer go out of the house other than for work unless I was with her or a friend came to pick her up. She could no longer trust her sense of balance; shopping alone became unfeasible.

Once in a while there were days when she could not get to work; I would leave her apartment early in the morning while she was still in bed, I would kiss her goodbye as she dozed, I would write her a love note, and I would lock the door behind me. It was not until she tried to get up that she would realize there was something wrong. When we spoke a little later in the day she would tell me she was still in bed unable to function properly and unable to endure the walk to the car, the drive to work, and then walking from the parking lot to her desk. It was simply too much to even contemplate leaving the house on days like these.

On other occasions, and these were the ones that worried me the most, she would fall in her apartment and would not be able to get up for hours on end, unable to reach the phone to call me; her body would literally shut down. Her arms became too weak to pull her along the floor to get to the phone; she would lie there until, somehow, someway, her body 're-booted' itself and she managed to make the call.

- What did you do, Angel? - I asked.

- Just lay there and waited - She replied.

The first time she told me this had happened, I sat at the other end of the line, silent tears welling in my eyes for her as she described herself lying in a heap, helpless and desperate, yet seemingly resigned to the event. For some reason I never allowed her to know how saddened I was by her ordeal; there was just something in the way she spoke of these things that made me realize she did not want or need me to be sad. It was important that we maintained an air of relative normalcy within these frightening and inconclusive parameters.

Then came the day I called her work in the late morning, but they said she had not come in; I quickly called her home - she did not answer either the landline or her cell. I began to worry and after repeated efforts to reach her I decided to drive up and make certain she was okay. It was unlike her to not pick up one of her phones when I called or to at least to call me back. When I arrived at her apartment I knocked on the door but heard nothing. I knocked again, harder. Nothing. I let myself in. Normally, I would never have done this, but I knew something was wrong.

How Angels Die - A Confession

I called out.

- Angel?

I heard a faint

- I'm back here.

I rushed to her bedroom in the back of the apartment and I found Jemma on the floor, helpless, dried tears on her cheeks.

- Angel. Oh my God! - I exploded - What happened? Are you okay? I'm so sorry.

As I spoke I knelt down and lifted her up into my arms and carried her to the bathroom. It was not a dignified scene. She had clearly been lying there for a while and had not been able to hold in her basic needs. The smell was powerful; the situation was devastating. I placed her on the toilet seat and turned on the shower; I picked her up again and carried her, fully clothed, to the warm water. She did not speak; she just let me take control. I did not speak, there was nothing to say.

I stepped into the shower with her and I began to strip her naked, piling her soiled clothes in the corner of the shower, and I washed her. As I cleaned her, her dead weight became too much for me to hold so I sat her down on the shower floor and I slumped down next to her letting the steam and water wash over us both. I was exhausted, emotionally and physically, from what I had just seen and done.

I wanted to burst into tears. I began to feel the warmth rush into my eyes. I looked at Jemma to see if she was okay, dreading what I was about to see. She looked across at me with a sideways glance, her face lit up, and she began to giggle.

- You are so crazy - She said.

- I am?

- Look at you. You're still dressed - She carried on as she giggled at me.

I smiled at her, took her face in my hands and kissed her lips with all my might.

- I love you so fucking much, Angel.

- I know - She replied - I know.

And there we sat; soaking wet. Two drenched lovers in the midst of our own personal hell; and even then, in the depths of the situation that we had to conquer, even then, Jemma managed to find a reason to smile.

I could not allow myself to think of what she was going through despite all that we were managing together. If I ever wallowed in her pain it would affect me so physically that I wanted to break down.

How Angels Die - A Confession

I felt so helpless in so many ways. It was a disease that had no rhyme nor reason - inflicted on someone so sweet and mild that the cruelty of it all was too much for my heart to cope with. I was completely and utterly at a loss for what to do because I was aware that no matter what, I could not take away her daily struggle, I could not make her trauma any easier; I could only sympathize, empathize, and be there to support her when she was hit by another merciless thunderbolt.

The position I was left in was untenable. I wanted, so badly, to be able to remove her from the situation she was in - I wanted to 'make everything better' - I wanted to whisk her away and start all over again.

There was a beastliness to this disease, an inoperable and consequential effect that left me as an observer, watching the one I loved struggle to fight back against an enemy she could not see, while I stood on the sidelines, my arm outstretched, hoping she would take my hand and be free from the fight she had not asked for, free from the attacks she had not instigated and free from the strikes of the MS that caused her to collapse under the strain of their piercing aim.

Yet, as many times as she took my hand, and as often as I tried to support her, the disease would fight back even harder and she would once again succumb to the relentlessness of the onslaught. Dwelling on these thoughts only served to weaken me, to drag me into a depth of melancholy that was simply detrimental to both of us, and so, I adopted Jemma's strength and Jemma's mantra; I denied myself the luxury of pity and I overcame my bitter sadness by counter-balancing that pain with love. I eradicated the anguish by displaying only love, by giving myself fully to her cause and by knowing that even if it was only helping her slightly then it was worth every ounce of the struggle.

Without her knowing, I vowed to be with her more often, to make sure that there would never be more than a two or three hour period when we would have no contact.

I called her immediately after my workout everyday to wish her good morning and to make sure she was up and on her way to work; in this way I could check up on her health without appearing to be prying. During the day I would stop by the Gallery or I would call her with little anecdotes as an excuse to see how she was. Whatever I could do to maintain contact, I would, because I wanted to be sure that I had at least some idea of her whereabouts just in case she fell and was paralyzed with overwhelming weakness again.

On the days that she did not feel up to the journey to work and a full day in the Gallery, I might return to her apartment if she wanted me to and we would spend the day together. If I was traveling, which I sometimes had to do because now I was involved in designing clothes in Brazil and China for sale in the USA, I would make arrangements to have friends contact her regularly and I would call just as often as usual to keep abreast of her health. I did all of this without her ever knowing my real intentions, for, despite our closeness and despite my understanding of everything she was going through, Jemma was, in her own quiet way, insistent she would be "fine" - even if I saw otherwise.

I felt it was my duty to keep up this charade of compliance - to be aware of everything that she was dealing with whilst mentioning nothing of what I knew unless she mentioned it first. Only then, would we discuss the terrible situation she faced. If she had known how worried I was she would have felt guilty for putting me through those emotions and she might not have been honest with me when we spoke.

It was essential to the delicate balance of our communication that I did not allow her to feel any pressure from me or to feel any fear in telling me how she was. It was as if I was luring her into a false sense of ease in order that I could help her without her feeling that I was a watch-guard analyzing her every move. It was in her character to avoid being reliant upon someone else, to avoid being a responsibility, although, for my part I was more than willing to do whatever I could. Even with her strong desire not to make any unnecessary drama, the reality of her plight became unavoidable.

How Angels Die - A Confession

- The worst part about it is that I don't actually feel any pain, so it doesn't make any sense to me - She would say.

- Apart from where you have fallen and hurt yourself - I would point out.

- I know, but it's not like the MS is painful. My balance is getting worse by the day, though. It worries me a bit.

The next time she visited the doctor, some weeks later, she told him that the weakness in her legs was affecting her ability to walk and that her episodes were becoming more frequent and severe. It was decided that she should advance her medication from pills to injections. These newer steroids were thought to be a far more powerful ally against the onslaught of the MS.

Even so, there were still times when I grew frustrated with her regarding her health. I felt that she was sometimes giving up, allowing the disease to control her, accepting her 'fate', and in these moments I would voice my opinions.

- Angel - I would begin - How about we get you onto some sort of exercise regime; something easy that will maintain your muscle strength, something to keep you in relatively good shape.

She would be silent for a second before replying.

- It's not that easy, I don't feel like doing anything most of the time.

I would continue to push.

- That's not a very good way to look at it. Even a couple of times a week, some stretching, some yoga moves, some light weights; it would all help.

Her frustration would grow.

- I just don't feel like it, Monkey - She retorted - I know it will do no good anyway.

- No you don't. You have to at least try.

- Do I? What's the point? It's all going to lead to the same conclusion in the end, my body will give up and I will be left helpless.

This would upset me.

- It doesn't have to be that way. You have to think positively; we can overcome anything if we put our mind to it, we can fix ourselves if we want to. And we should get you onto a better diet too; you are eating and drinking too much sugar.

- Please stop going on at me - She would conclude - I don't want to worry about everything I do; I do my best and I will let the rest happen in whatever way it does. Anyway, like you said, it doesn't matter in the long run, does it? Aren't you the one that said that to me?

My own argument thrown in my face. I suppose I deserved it in some way, I was so opinionated about certain things that I was bound to get caught out in the end.

- Okay - I would finalize - But please promise me you won't just give up.

She would greet this request with silence and the abruptness of our disagreement would always disappoint me. I could not make her better without her help. I could not fight without the fear of being cast aside. So, once again, I let her have it her way...

13

My time in the USA had been divided into three phases - tourist, illegal alien and legal resident alien. The latter of these three was based upon the fact that I was a talented individual who had a unique ability to perform a task that no American citizen could compete with. (I know, it makes no sense to me either).

It was a tenuous position to be in, resident legal alien; a juxtaposition of insecurity and comfort that allowed me to remain on American soil provided I had an employer, or rather a Sponsor, who regarded my talents as essential to their business, a talent that could not be found in any other United States citizen. I had achieved this by convincing a model agent to take me on despite my less than stellar photographs and campaigns from my time in England; but since my arrival and my consequent visa approval I had not been to one casting or secured a single job.

I was spending my savings on recording as many songs as I could in the hope of securing a record deal that always seemed to elude me. Luckily I was making quite good money from investing in the stock market which was in its heyday; but none of this would endear me to the American immigration authorities as most of my assets were offshore in British bank accounts and my income in the USA was, as far as the immigration law was concerned, non-existent. Time was running out on this little ruse of mine, and I knew that soon I would have to either get a Green Card or get out.

When I had initially landed in California, I went to an immigration lawyer in the San Fernando Valley whose first words were

- Do you know anyone that would marry you?

I was flabbergasted for a second, but managed to utter

- Yes. But not anybody that I would propose to.

He looked at me across his desk and said in the most prophetic voice he could muster

- Then this will not be easy.

Unfortunately, he was right. And so now, here I was, six years later, needing a hand to acquire a Green Card if I was to be able to stay in my new found home.

As a citizen of the United States, one has no idea how complicated and fraught with danger this process is.

How Angels Die - A Confession

Every 't' must be crossed, every 'i' must be dotted and even then the outcome has no guarantee. The horror stories I had heard were almost enough to make me give up right then and there, but California held a particularly special place in my heart and now my life, so I was not about to leave without some sort of effort.

As much as I tried to think of other ways, and as much as I thought of myself as a unique talent, a zero income balance is not very impressive in one's chosen career and what was important was that I was seen as a productive and irreplaceable member of society; this was a tough one to prove as I was neither.

And so, one day, much to my shame and very much against everything I stood for with regards to matrimony, I plucked up the courage to ask Jemma for a monumental favor.

- Angel? - I said hesitantly.

- Yes, Monkey - She replied nonchalantly.

- You know that my visa is about to expire and I have no real means of staying here once it does? - I hurriedly spurted.

- Yes, Monkey - She replied knowingly.

- Well, do you think you would marry me so that I could get my Green Card?

Romantic, right? It came out completely wrong. But, I suppose, it got the point across.

She paused for a few seconds. She still did not look at me or even avert her eyes away from the television that neither of us were watching although we were both looking at it.

- Is there not another way? - She asked, pointedly.

- Not that I can see. It's the only way that is a near certainty. Although it is illegal, I should warn you of that.

She paused for a few seconds and then she looked me straight in the eye.

- I'm sorry, Monkey. No. I can't do it. I don't want to get married. And I don't want to go to prison.

I was, in all honesty, shocked. I did not think she would refuse me, but I understood completely.

- Okay - I said - That's a problem. But I get it. Plan B then.

- What's Plan B? - She asked.

- Don't have one - I replied.

All I knew for certain was that it was September, and I had until March of the next year to work out a plan of action that would allow me to stay in California. If the worst came to the worst, I thought, I will just stay and never leave US soil, as they would probably never catch me anyway - whoever 'they' were.

I was now faced with a two-fold problem. If I was deported, the life I knew would be ripped away from me, the hard work I had put into my music, my clothes design and my California life would be gone - this, I could handle. But what about Jemma? Who would look after her? If I was not able to be here, close to her, then she would be all alone, facing this battle without support, struggling to survive. When I thought about this, my throat tightened, my heart beat faster, my adrenaline soared and my instinct to scream was hard to control. But, control it I did. For the moment. For Jemma. In the hope that I would somehow be able to stay and love her.

I did not mention marriage again. I knew how she felt about it, it was the same way I felt, and I knew there was no point in pushing the point. She had been very clear with her answer and I did not want to annoy her, or disgrace myself by pleading with her about 'our' situation. Something would come to light, I felt sure of that, and until then, I would just keep thinking positively and actively about a favorable outcome.

I took my chances, and as chance would have it, chance gave me a chance.

14

Jemma's mother came to visit with her husband that November which proved to be the catalyst for my little miracle. Jemma had said to me before their arrival

- I have told my mom that you're only here for one night and then you're out of town so you don't have to come to dinner every night while they are here. I love you too much to put you through that.

I had not yet met her mother, even after all these years, and so this was to be the big reveal. Jemma was concerned I would get roped into days and nights of parental care even she found hard to deal with, and so she had devised her little white lie to protect me from imminent madness.

- Thanks, Angel - I replied - I appreciate that.

When we had spoken of it in the past, she would sometimes ask me why I did not want to meet her mother.

- Because I'm dating you, not her, and I'd rather avoid the boring chit chat if possible.

How Angels Die - A Confession

- But I met your mum - She would reply.

- I know - I would say - But my mum is cool and you told me that your mom is not.

Jemma laughed. She knew I was right.

I finally met her mother on a Thursday night in November. Generally, I find parents easy to handle, if a little dull to negotiate. I know that they want the meeting to be comfortable too and so I do my best to ensure that the conversation is as light-hearted and as familiar as possible, which seems to work for all concerned; I have found that if you act like an old friend, then they seem to think you are.

We had an early dinner accompanied by Christina and her new boyfriend, Anthony, and then afterwards we had drinks in their hotel suite. Her mother was a very demure lady, her husband very precise. They were a quiet, homebody couple who had their methods of living and rarely broke the routine, even when they traveled. I liked them very much and at the end of the evening, we all mentioned that it would be a pleasure to meet again. As we drove away from the hotel, Jemma said

- Thank you for doing that. I tried to keep you away from it as long as possible, but I think the time had come when the excuses had run out.

- I know, Angel, but they were very sweet and kind and it's good to at last have met them after having heard so much. As nice as they are, I completely see your opinion on them and understand why you feel as you do.

Jemma had always found her mother to be a little too inquisitive and sometimes her mother fell into a forced act of ignorance about things that Jemma knew she knew; it was just a way to try to make her children feel intelligent, but rather than endearing herself to the twins, it simply aggravated them. Added to this, her mother had become overtly Christian since she met her second husband, Bob, and this infuriated Jemma more than anything, because she felt it was so fake. I had noticed these traits during the evening, but only because they had been pointed out to me beforehand. In general I found her mother and step father to be very mild, upstanding, pleasant people.

As it happened, Jemma suffered a slight relapse during her mother's visit. The MS was playing up and she had to spend a couple of days at home. I visited her during those days, but left before the family arrived in the evenings as I was supposed to be out of town. The pressure of entertaining at home proved to be too much for Jemma, and so on the Sunday night she did not see her family at all, she stayed in bed and convalesced. They left the next day.

- Having them round to my house was so intrusive - She said - They kept re-arranging my things, looking through my life, questioning everything; it really took a toll on me. I just couldn't deal with it. They mean well, I know that, but they don't get me at all.

It was not long after this visit that Jemma began to ask me about my status in the USA.

- So, getting married is the best way for you to get a Green Card?

- Yes. It's a little risky, but because we are of similar age, background and race, it will appear to be on the up and up. We don't have to live together, we can have two homes - I reassured her.

- And then you would be in charge of my estate and my life, should anything happen to me, right?

- Yes. Why?

- I don't know, but since my mom was here, I have come to the conclusion that my family have no idea about what I want. They don't care what I want, they only see things the way they see them and I don't think they would respect my wishes if I needed them to. The amount of times I have asked my mom not to do things which she then does despite my requests is worrying to me. I don't really trust her to listen...

As she spoke, I realized it was the first time she had verbalized her fear of being dependent upon someone else in case the MS took over her body and did not relinquish control. The tone she emitted was one of acceptance; it was as if an inner-understanding had been reached that she would, one day, become immobile should the MS continue unabated.

Jemma was adept at saying a great deal with very few words; she had an inherent ability to leave a conversation at the exact point where one could conclude the rest of her meaning in one's own head.

I mulled over her words, disregarding the advantage marriage would have for my status. I decided to let her think about it, I did not pressure her at all. This was for her to decide.

And then, one Friday morning, early in December, Jemma called me while I was at home in Laguna.

- What are you doing on Tuesday? - She asked.

- Nothing - I replied - Why?

- Wanna get married?

- Are you joking?

- No.

- Then, yes - I said as I burst into laughter.

How Angels Die - A Confession

After we put the phone down, I called my lawyer and asked him how to get married with as little fuss as possible.

- Go to the Santa Clara Courthouse in the morning after 11AM. You don't need an appointment, just two rings - He said.

Jemma and I did not talk about it over the next three days; it had been decided. She had managed to get the day off work and there was nothing more to say, so, on that Tuesday morning, we woke up early and prepared ourselves for our wedding day.

When morning arrived Jemma did not feel well and the idea of driving two hours from Hollywood filled her with dread - especially as she needed to use the bathroom more regularly than normal and sometimes the need arose without warning.

It took us a full half hour to finally get out the door because Jemma wanted to be certain she was prepared for the long journey. Her mind began to rule her body in these situations and so she was frequently paralyzed into thinking that she needed the bathroom when she did not. I waited quietly, patiently and sympathetically as she stalled our exit and I tried to calm her anxiety with my understanding.

Once we were in the car I drove as far and as fast as I could. Even so, Jemma still needed three bathroom breaks. Sadly, one of them was in a parking lot as she could not make it to the nearest restaurant bathroom in time. I stood guard over her, doing my best to ease her anguish and embarrassment, trying to help her get back to a positive place before we resumed our journey. She was amazingly resilient about all of it and did not make a bigger deal than necessary; such was her way. After each stop we resumed the journey without discussion or analysis; she did not want to talk and so I respected her silence.

We arrived at the courthouse around 11AM and signed ourselves in, filling out the required paperwork and waiting our turn. Half an hour later, we were in front of the relevant officiary, in a small chapel-like room, exchanging vows and rings.

It was the line 'til death do us part' that most resonated with me. I knew full well that Jemma had agreed to marry me as an insurance policy against her family keeping her alive despite her overwhelming desire to be "put out of her misery" should there be a remote possibility of doing so.

- My mother has become so 'holier than thou' since she married Bob. I want the decisions I make, or the ones made for me, to be practical, not based on Jesus Christ Our Lord and Savior - She had commented - My mother is incapable of doing what I ask of her, even the simplest things like not buying me ridiculous gifts, and so I know she will not respect my wishes when it comes down to more serious issues, she will do what she wants to do and that won't be what I want or ask her to do.

We left the courthouse and walked out into the blazing sun as husband and wife. We held hands and kissed on the steps. There are no photographs of the occasion or even of the day; this was simply a time for us to bond so that we knew we could remain together and be there for each other in times of uncertainty. I suppose that is one of the reasons marriage was originally invented - a protection mechanism against the outside forces that we have so little control over. This union meant the law could no longer separate us or over-ride our wishes; we were now a team, fully legal and fully capable of being together without interference.

Well, almost.

I spoke to my lawyer again and found out that I now had to go through the rigamarole of obtaining a Parole Letter which would allow me to go in and out of the country without being arrested or turned away. I then had to apply for the Green Card, which required Jemma and I to prove our marital status was for real - not just a way of avoiding deportation. We had to have joint bank accounts, bills and other points of reference that allowed the Immigration & Naturalization Service to tick all the boxes before we could have the Green Card interview. This was a long process and sometimes the interview could be two years away.

How Angels Die - A Confession

During this time I had to miss one Green Card appointment as I was in Paris for a clothing trade show and when I returned home there was a letter on my doorstep which informed me that I was now an illegal alien and should leave the country immediately. This sent me into panic stations and I called my lawyer again, who reassured me it was a standard letter and he would sort it out for me; in the end it required us starting the whole process again which cost me another five thousand dollars.

The Green Card meeting was finally set for the following November, nearly a year after our marriage. We drove to downtown LA and I dropped Jemma off outside the Federal Building before parking the car. Her mobility was terrible at this stage and I had to place her carefully on a bench before leaving her. I then returned and had to support her as we stood in the security line that stretched around the block. When we finally entered the building, we went to the sixth floor and waited for our lawyer-of-the-day to arrive, which she did in good time.

As she looked through our paperwork, the taciturn lawyer commented

- You really don't have enough here to warrant a Green Card. There is less here than in most three month marriages. I am not sure I can make this work for you, but I will try.

She was right. Jemma and I were both very resistant to the idea of a standard marriage. We felt it would only hinder our easy lifestyle and so, despite our marital status, we had done little to change our arrangements. We had only a few bills in joint names, one bank account, a car payment and not much else other than photographs, and even these were few and far between because Jemma disliked having her photograph taken at the best of times. As the lawyer spoke, my heart sank and my fear level rose immeasurably. Had all of this been a waste of time?

- Now - The lawyer continued - Only answer the question asked. If she asks you if you have a car, say "Yes". Don't tell her what make or color of car unless she asks for those details. Do you understand me?

We both replied in the affirmative and sat there, holding hands, our palms beginning to perspire as we realized how serious this whole situation now was.

Ten minutes later, the immigration officer called us in. I walked with Jemma, slowly. I held her arm, and then our lawyer made a point of stating that Jemma had MS, which we both felt was highly inappropriate although we said nothing, there was nothing we could say; I suppose she had her reasons.

When we reached the tiny office, we sat down with our backs to the wall a foot or two from the desk. I was in the middle, Jemma to my left, the lawyer to my right, the immigration officer on the other side of the desk. She was a young Hispanic woman who looked calmly over the paperwork.

- And so - She said, looking at Jemma - What's it like being married to a model?

Jemma laughed a little and then said

- It's okay. He doesn't get too big headed about it.

The officer smiled and then looked at me.

- I knew you had to be something out of the ordinary, especially with the way you dress.

I did not quite know what to say. I had dressed as conservatively as I knew how - no tattoos were showing, tortoise shell clear-lensed glasses instead of my usual sunglass framed pair, brown leather shoes, chocolate brown slacks, a cream shirt and a tan jacket. I suppose I was still a little too English for LA.

After a second or so, I smiled and said

- It makes up for my face.

She smiled politely back at me - she did not laugh as I had hoped. Her eyes flicked to Jemma and she looked down at the paperwork again. I felt our lawyer shift uncomfortably in her seat. The immigration officer finally looked up at Jemma again.

How Angels Die - A Confession

- And what do your family think of him?

- They love him - She lied - He makes them laugh and they're big fans of the English accent.

The officer then asked a range of questions; how long ago did we meet? How did we meet? What were her siblings names? Where were my parents? Why did we have two homes and did we plan on having children? We took all the questions in our stride and answered them as instructed by our lawyer. We came across as a loving and easy-going couple. Jemma and I held hands the whole time. Finally, the officer looked at the ring on my wedding finger; it was a diamond encrusted horse shoe shape.

- I really like your choice of ring - She said - Very interesting.

Jemma, without missing a beat, held up her left hand and placed it on the desk.

- I have the same one - She pointed out.

- How cool! - Exclaimed the officer - Those are the coolest rings I've ever seen.

She then carried on studying the paperwork and a minute later, after having glanced at our lawyer, she declared

How Angels Die - A Confession

- I see no problem with your application, I will just have to run a check on the terrorist watch list and you should be fine. I would imagine you will have your Green Card within ninety days.

I wanted to jump up and punch the air, to laugh at our lawyer, to hug the immigration officer, to kiss Jemma all over her face, on her lips, her ears, everywhere...

But I did not.

I sat there, stone faced and said

- Thank you.

Our lawyer said the same and then we all got up, shook hands and the three of us walked out of another door in the office that led back into the waiting area. As we stepped into the room filled with chairs and a scattering of people, our lawyer said, a little too loudly

- You are very, very lucky. I would never have granted that application.

I wanted to smother her mouth and put a black hood over her head for being so unsubtle...

But I did not.

I smiled and thanked her. She carried on

- And I have never in my life heard an immigration officer say the word 'cool'.

I think she was almost offended that we had broken the mould and got away with it; she seemed a little put out that the rules had not been followed and we had still managed to pass the test. We both smiled at her now and thanked her again for her time. I helped Jemma slowly back to the elevator and outside to the car.

Once we were in the car and driving home, we began to talk.

- What a nightmare - Jemma said.

- You were brilliant, Angel. The gem was when you held up your horse shoe ring. I think that sealed the deal.

- Me too. Well, thank God that's over with. It's so ridiculous that we had to endure all of that just so you can stay here and I can have my wishes adhered to.

- I know, especially considering the British and Americans won the Second World War together and now I can't even live here without begging; and as for the ridiculous laws governing final wishes, I almost understand why gays want to get married. The whole thing is so stupid.

How Angels Die - A Confession

The fear and concern of deportation had suddenly been lifted; I was going to be a permanent resident of the USA with the ability to look after My Angel through her darkest times. This elation was hard to grasp because it was not really a physical prize one could hold and lift up above one's head. It was primarily emotional. Jemma was sick, perhaps dying, and I had been terrified of not being able to help her. Now, all of a sudden, I felt free, I felt powerful, I felt significant and capable and full of love despite the rocky times I knew we had ahead of us.

- I have to write a living will - Jemma stated out of the blue - just in case something does happen. It means you can turn off the machine if they try to keep me alive too long and they won't try to resuscitate me should my heart stop beating.

- This is a little morbid, isn't it? - I commented.

- But necessary - She replied - We did this for the right reasons, didn't we, Monkey?

- Yes we did, Angel. Love is the worst reason to get married, it screws up everything! - I joked.

We both laughed loudly, our laughter was filled with joy, we were joined together by law, we were holding hands, we were in love; nobody else we knew had a clue about what we had just done, and there was no reason they should ever find out.

I squeezed Jemma's soft and delicate hand and we drove back to her apartment in Hollywood where a different kind of existence united us.

15

Initially, injecting the steroids was a semi-effective antidote - they would help Jemma maintain her balance and allow her to walk more easily for a few days so the pain of administering them all by herself was almost worth it, but every so often, she would feel quite sick for a day or two afterwards.

- Sometimes I wonder if this is all worth it - She said - whichever way I turn I'm dealing with something annoying and whatever I do doesn't seem to cure the problem.

She did not want an answer at the time; she just wanted to make the point. I understood completely. She had this facade of strength, this determination to overcome whatever it was that hindered her life; but to watch her as she battled through the difficulties she was presented with was agonizing for me. I was pleased that the steroids helped her walk without falling so frequently and I was glad to see her stick to the routine of injections no matter how much she would rather have taken a pill.

How Angels Die - A Confession

Every three days she would sit upright on the sofa in front of the TV with her legs exposed, the syringe in her hand and her thumb on the plunger, the needle hovering over the bare skin. She would then tell herself that she would inject her leg when the commercials began; when the commercials began she would tell herself that she would do it when they ended. It carried on like this for hours sometimes, shows would start and finish, the news came and went, but in the end, the long needle pricked and slid under the skin and the fluid entered her body enabling her some respite from the worries of falling down and hurting herself. The first time she injected herself she had asked me to be with her.

- I don't know if I can do this - She said.

- Do you want me to do it, Angel?

- No. Not yet. I want to try. I have to learn.

- Okay. You just let me know. Do you want me to hold your other hand or your shoulder, something to reassure you?

- Yes, please. That might help.

She wavered for a very long time between injecting herself and asking me to do it; she could not quite come to a decision. I remember the angst I felt - fearing that she would not be able to do it - which would leave me to inject her. I was not sure I would be able to go through with it either. Even so, I pretended that I had no problem injecting her if she wanted me to, despite my reservations. Luckily, she was far braver than me.

When she finally became adept at injecting herself with the old fashioned needle and syringe, she was sent an injector that hid the needle and simply required her to place the tube on her leg and press a button on the top. Not seeing the needle made a world of difference to the process - but unfortunately it made no difference to the effect.

Over time, the bruises from the injections became painful and the location of entry had to change. Her skin did not heal quickly anymore and as her health deteriorated; the steroids became less and less effective.

By now, a few months later, there was visible bloating around her face and neck, her skin became pale, and on top of this the steroids would also make her feel very sick nearly every time she took them. She had a choice: feel sick and be able to walk, or feel well and be immobile. It was a choice that I would not wish on anyone, least of all the person I loved most - particularly when it was someone as lovely as Jemma.

When she felt sick, she could not eat and she felt miserable; when she felt normal, she fell over and bruised herself so she had swollen and sore knees that left bloodstains on the floor where she landed. Her body did not communicate the collapse to her mind quickly enough and so she rarely had the where-with-all to break the crashing descent that would follow.

It was heartbreaking to see her cuts and her bruises, to witness her muscles slowly atrophy, to observe her bravery as she struggled on without ever saying a negative word. My love and respect for her was already immense and grew immeasurably as she faced her demons without complaint, without self-pity, only with strength and acceptance.

As things became worse, she ended up having to sit on the floor of the shower because her legs became too weak for her to stand for any period of time and then, adding insult to injury, she lost the ability to know when she needed to relieve herself - sometimes it was every five minutes and other times not at all, even if she thought she had to. This was made more acute when she worried. Going to work or going shopping would invariably lead to her feeling panicked and uncomfortable which made everyday life almost unbearable.

When we walked anywhere, I would have to constantly hold her arm to support her because she had become so weak and wobbly - people would think she was drunk and once in a while they would even make inappropriate and accusatory comments as she went towards the car with the keys in her hand. I know she felt the stares and sometimes heard the unkind words. It must have been monumentally demoralizing and acutely upsetting for someone as sensitive as Jemma to be the victim of these idle remarks.

Being by her side, I experienced many of the worst moments, and although I put a brave face on it all for her sake, I could tell the time was coming when she would have to give up work, when the journey alone would be over-bearing and the practicality of walking around the Gallery would be impossible.

At home, she began to use a metal walker to help her get around if I was not there to carry her. The steroids were no longer working and nor was her body, despite every effort she was making to give herself a fighting chance.

- I wonder if it's the pollution that's making me ill - She said one day.

- I guess it could be - I replied - I know of people who move to LA and are seriously affected by it. Do you think you should spend some time back in Denver, get some fresh air?

- No. I don't want to go back there, it would depress me and I would feel uncomfortable. I want to stay here, there's nowhere else that I want to go.

How Angels Die - A Confession

We researched the possibility of pollution playing a part in her illness but it seemed that MS was usually associated with colder climates - the East Coast of America has a far higher instance of MS than the West Coast, and Jemma was originally brought up in Massachusetts. This information made sure she remained in LA. She preferred the heat even though it did not exactly help her in some ways - especially at the height of summer. But I was glad that she would remain near, where I could at least be a sounding board and a support for her, where she could maintain her independence and a sense of normalcy.

She looked into her medical plan and, after some deliberation, she finally spoke to her boss about the problems she was having. He was very understanding and told her not to worry about her job; he said she should work on getting herself as healthy as she could and he mentioned to her that there would always be a position at the Gallery available to her.

As the months progressed, along with the disease becoming more rampant, she ended up having to take more and more sick days and began to feel guilty about being such an irregular employee. I could see her spirit becoming resigned to the fact that she was fighting a losing battle. Her invisible and intangible enemy was slowly and methodically winning the war of attrition which would eventually control her body - despite her courage and determination. Although she kept smiling, her demeanor changed, she became a little more introverted and a little quieter.

How Angels Die - A Confession

There were times I would walk into the room and she would be sitting on the sofa in her own little world, distracted by the enormity of her battle, contemplating the options and the changes she faced. I would watch her for minutes at a time, wishing I could do something but realizing that she needed to come to her own conclusions because she was the only one who could work out the right answer for her. As I stood quietly, still, my whole being would ache with love for her. My heart would feel her pain and when I could bear it no longer, I would walk over to her, break her trance and hold her in my arms for a long, long time, quietly enveloping her, loving her. As I did this, I could sense that she was distracted, a little distant, turning all the possibilities around in her head.

I would visit the Gallery regularly when she was able to work, as I always had, although we no longer went for lunches because she found it hard to walk more than a few feet. I would sit next to her for a while and we would talk as we held hands and drank a tea, a coffee or even a hot chocolate.

Somedays I would stop by a few times just to surprise her and hopefully break up the monotony of sitting at her desk; I was always greeted with a joyful smile and a warm kiss. I became quite friendly with some of the sales staff as well who were very kind and generous. They could tell that something was wrong despite Jemma's privacy, and even though I am sure they wanted to ask questions, they helped her when they could and kept an eye on her at other times.

How Angels Die - A Confession

All forms of movement were becoming overwhelming for Jemma - even walking to her boss's office was a feat she avoided as much as possible. In the evenings, she expressed how useless she was beginning to feel and how difficult it was to do the job required of her, as simple as it had seemed only a few months before.

- I think I might have to stop going to work - She finally said - I don't feel right about being paid for a job I can't really do anymore.

- And if you get better, you can always go back, right?

- Yes, that door is always open. In the meantime I would get disability, but it wouldn't be much.

- Don't worry about the money, we will get you whatever you need, whenever you need it - I replied - I just want you to be as comfortable as possible.

I could see her visibly relax when she saw I was not fazed by this monumental decision that would change our dynamic immeasurably. I think it gave her the ability to look beyond where she was now, stuck in a spiral of fear that every morning would bring - the drive to work had become intolerable and walking unaided was almost impossible for her on many days. Perhaps, given time and rest, she might now find a way to overcome her physical issues. We talked about all of this regularly for a few weeks until the decision was made.

Finally, after six and a half years, the MS won its first battle against Jemma and she reluctantly left work on disability.

In some ways this was a good thing, it released her from the pressures of the daily grind and therefore released her from a great deal of worry. In other ways, it simply clarified and magnified her disease and the havoc it had scattered and reaped in her life. She was unable to enjoy her freedom, she was not mobile anymore, and the days seemed very long when she had so little to do, because now, she was essentially housebound.

16

Although this new situation was not ideal and despite the occasional 'mishap' with Jemma, nothing seemed to hinder or disrupt the joy we felt with each other, and we continued appreciating our special love even though we were at her apartment most of the time when we were together.

As we had promised ourselves, we had been sky-diving every year up until now and on our way home we always gorged ourselves on Krispy Kremes as a bonus treat for our bravery. The last time we went, Jemma's tandem instructor insisted on doing some aerobatical tricks once they had finished the free fall and had pulled the parachute open - he was spinning her round and around which made her feel queazy.

- I wouldn't do that - She warned him - I'm about to throw up.

- No you won't, don't worry - Came his reply.

Less than a minute later Jemma kept her word. I had already vacated my parachute and was waiting for her on the ground, watching proudly as she prepared for the final descent; but as she landed I was greeted with a surprise, I could see the evidence of the aerobatics all over her and all over the instructor's jumpsuit. Once they had unclipped from each other, she got the giggles. She was so embarrassed and so incredulous over what had happened; she did not stop laughing until we were on the freeway driving home.

- I warned him. I did warn him - She kept saying as she suppressed another outburst of laughter.

These adventurous times, our annual trip to go sky-diving, our beach trips, our travels, were now memories or impossibilities for us and I was saddened by them because they were just that, memories; a life that was behind us. Gone. Jemma could no longer live the life she once enjoyed and I could no longer put my heart into doing those things without her.

From the very beginning of our relationship we spoke every day, more often than was probably healthy, but we were fortunate enough to know that regular communication was an essential part of any successful, long term relationship, as much as we were aware that space was also an essential ingredient of that same situation.

We had invented more affectionate nicknames than were necessary and over time they all morphed into pretty much meaningless drivel only to be understood by the two of us and only to be used in private. There were full-on alter egos existing in our sphere that managed to become part of our peculiar little 'family' - sometimes Jemma would banish these characters to faraway lands where they were without any form of transportation and so could not return (or at least that was what she told me). That was when I knew she had had enough and so we invented someone new; whether it was a mouse, a bratty child or a cheeky monkey, they all managed to find a way into her heart before their eventual and inevitable 'displacement'. We would reminisce regularly and we would always laugh at the ridiculous outcomes of these imaginary characters.

Over the years, I had traveled quite a lot for work. I was now designing and selling women's clothing full time - everything from lingerie to denim - and so Brazil, Hong Kong, China, Europe, New York & Las Vegas were all regular trips for me.

When I was not close, I naturally worried about Jemma. I would call as often as possible, but in the end I knew I was powerless when away and so had to simply deal with the situation as best I could from afar - she never gave me cause to worry, even though I am quite sure she had plenty to deal with that I was unaware of.

I ended up buying her a monkey teddy bear so she would have something to cuddle at night while I was in distant lands. When I was home, she would invariably use him as an excuse for why all the chocolate had been eaten during the day, or she would mention his desire to see me when she wanted me to come over; he was a regular little busy body. On more than one occasion I returned to her apartment to find Monkey sitting on the bed with his arms tightly crossed over his chest.

- He's a little upset with you - She would say, smirking - He says you've neglected him and so he ate all the ice cream.

And that was that, no ice cream for me, with nobody to take it out on but a stuffed animal; it was quite uncanny how she made him look almost guilty with his head bowed low and his eyes looking down. Her sense of humor was very playful and natural, and rather than quash my alarming energy for invention, she would allow me to play out my craziness whilst adding her own variations for her apparent amusement. Hence my nickname - Monkey. She was so good with me, so patient, and despite my sometime irrational lunacy, she always managed to see the funny side of these antics which became an important part of our daily lives - the light relief that we needed as the other parts of our existence became more and more difficult.

Now that Jemma was at home, her disability began to take its toll on her mentally as well. She would spend the whole day inside, unable to get around with any ease - her friends and acquaintances were at work, and even if they were available she did not always feel up to socializing in her present condition - on most days, she would stay in her pajamas and she would settle down on the sofa in the morning watching MTV, followed by Ellen de Generes in the afternoons; in the early evenings it was the news programs or re-runs of shows she once enjoyed as a little girl.

Walking had become so difficult that even shoes would only serve to confuse her balance. She discarded footwear in favor of bare feet which meant that her feet now developed small cuts from where they would drag on the bamboo matting floor she had chosen when she first moved in to the apartment. The lack of movement only served to weaken her legs further. Her muscles began to atrophy, her body was slowly closing down and her world began to close down in response to the despondance she was beginning to feel. She no longer wanted to see or be seen by people - the change in her appearance would only serve to create pity and sympathy which were the two things she could not abide on any level.

Within a very short time of leaving work, the only people she did see were those that knew the rules: be happy and cheerful, do not wallow in the sadness of her prospects and do not stay too long.

- I just have this feeling of total and utter loss - She once said - I have lost everything that I was. I am not who I thought I would be anymore.

- But you're still beautiful, My Angel - I said - And you still have the brightest smile and the loveliest laugh.

- Thank you, Monkey - She replied - Thank you.

And, again, we left it at that; she did not discuss her situation. The comments she made were few and far between. I was accustomed to letting conversations on her state of mind stall at any moment, to be dropped by the wayside, the point made and nothing labored upon.

In the past month or so I had been hosting an outlandish fashion documentary for the UK; we only filmed a few days a week in LA, but whenever there was a break or a location change and there was some set up time required before I was next needed I would drive over to Jemma's to see her, perhaps fix her some lunch or bring her a cold drink. Just spending time with her was what it was really about, trying to liven up her day, so the long hours at home would pass more easily. If I was unable to visit I would call and talk to her between filming slots whenever possible.

The summer was beginning to heat up and the heat played havoc with her MS which made her immobility even more acute. The last time we went shopping together, we went to Sears and I bought her a portable air conditioning unit to ease the heat in her apartment. She kept it close to her throughout the day so the cool air would be flowing around her all the time to reduce the damaging effect of the heat on her limbs and consequently her mind. I lost count of the times she thanked me for it. Every time she did, it only served as a reminder of how precarious her health had become.

Because I had seen the slow degeneration of her abilities, and because we had spent so many years dealing with the painfully erratic progress of her illness, I knew exactly what Jemma wanted - to act as if things were normal.

I knew not to watch her if she managed to walk to the bathroom alone - nowadays it was always with the metal walker, it was always very slowly and it was always with difficulty. I knew not to dwell on any stumbles or falls that she might have when I was with her - I would simply help her up and let her carry on if she wanted to, or help her back to her seat. I ignored her bruises, or simply gave them a gentle kiss when I saw them, but always without verbal comment. I was on hand if she had an emergency and would carry her to the bathroom if she needed me. I did her housework whenever it was time and I would do her laundry too, I would make the bed, prepare the food and do the washing up.

- You don't have to do that, Monkey - She would say.

- But I like to, Angel. I can't help it.

How Angels Die - A Confession

She would laugh at me; knowing I was a bit of a neat freak, she just let it go, and even though it made her feel all the more helpless it was an inevitable part of maintaining the household and I knew she could not do it herself, so I did it with pleasure, for both of us.

I would also put some healthy snacks in the fridge so she could eat well without having to make too much effort, and when I went to the farmer's market I bought organic fruit and vegetables. She particularly loved cucumbers, she always said they were very refreshing - so I would get those whenever I could; I would slice them and leave them out for her to enjoy. I wanted to maintain a quality of life that she could appreciate even if she was in her home all the time. I was thankful that we had made so much effort in the beginning to make it as comfortable and elegant as possible; now, this was her world.

By this time I was spending every night with her. Fortunately, the filming for the television show had become sporadic, and so even on the days when I was working I was only away from her for a little while - and if I was not working, I would be with her for the whole day, taking it easy, keeping her amused, loving her, helping the time flow by. We did not discuss my moving in, that would have made it too formal; I just made sure to have enough clothes with me to cover a few days and then I would go home, swop them out and come back again. In this way it did not seem like I was imposing on her privacy or her freedom, yet I had become a permanent fixture in her home and in her bed so we could be close during the darkest hours.

She did not like to cuddle all night like she used to, the MS regularly over-heated her body and as I was always warm we spent most of our sleeping time simply holding hands or touching our feet together for a feeling of closeness. Sex had become more and more irregular; Jemma became ashamed of her body, and this, coupled with the slight discomfort she felt with heat and touch meant that we were far less physical than we had been in the preceeding years.

When I was not around, Christina would often come over with Anthony and they might all sit outside in the shade. He would jump in the pool, do trick dives and splash around in the water. He was an actor and a comedian who had a quick mind and a subdued yet rapid humor; he amused Jemma immensely.

Christina was becoming quite concerned for Jemma's well-being, but Jemma put on a brave face and gave little away. Although they were on good terms again, and had been for a while, Jemma had not forgotten Christina's previous antics and so kept a certain distance between them. Christina, for her part, seemed to have made a concerted effort to right the wrongs of the past - she was very caring for Jemma, sometimes went shopping for her, bought her treats and called regularly. Jemma looked forward to their visits, it was a different energy for her, and Anthony was a very respectful and kind person. I appreciated their concern and I valued their efforts; they were an important part of the equation. I was also glad to see Jemma enjoy outside company.

There was little time for her to be sad when I was around because we kept the energy lively and amusing, I was always talking in silly voices, discussing what to do with our latest 'family' member, play acting for her, allowing her to take ridiculous photographs of me so that she could laugh at them when I was not around, allowing the child in me to grow and flourish - not that it needed much encouragement - so her mind was occupied with the latest 'episode' of banality rather than anything more sinister.

Although we were both 'happy-go-lucky' on the exterior, we also had darker interiors that were not afraid to explore subjects that most people do not talk about with any honesty or regularity. We were not fatalistic per se, but we were perhaps a little too realistic. I am sure the views we batted back and forth are shared by very few, at least outwardly, but our ability to discuss them enabled us to handle a terrible situation and allowed us to exist without the regular boundaries one might be accustomed to. For, despite the attempts we made to keep our spirits high, and even though we did not dwell on the inevitability of her plight, the unavoidable truth was that her physical condition was worsening.

How Angels Die - A Confession

Starting with her feet, her inability to co-ordinate was spreading to her other limbs as well, almost as if rooms were having the lights turned out, and as each light faded we wondered which room would be next.

Her legs had now become consistently numb and unresponsive so that the lower half of her body was nothing more than a burden that prevented her from any form of self-transportation. Added to this was the way she felt about her appearance - because her muscles were not being used, they began to atrophy and lose the form they once had, and the bloating caused by the steroids, particularly around her neck, only made her feel worse. The stress of losing the ability to walk and then seeing her body deteriorate only placed further pressure on her mental strength, and knowing that she could do very little to repair the damage made the spiral of anguish all the more agonizing.

- Do you mind if I don't take off my pajama bottoms tonight? - She said one night.

- Of course not, Angel. Why?

- It's just the bruises and the cuts are so awful and my legs don't look like they used to. I feel very unattractive.

With that, she pulled back the sheet and struggled onto the bed. I helped her a little and then pulled the sheet over her, but I knew that her silence was telling me she was not in the mood to talk or to be fussed over.

I turned out her light, and as I climbed in next to her, I lay close and kissed her forehead. I put my arms around her and held her. She looked at me in the faded lights from the street - there was a sadness in her gaze, but the love she radiated was, as always, overwhelming.

- Goodnight, My Angel.

- Goodnight, Monkey... Thank you.

That was all she needed to say.

17

Because Jemma could feel herself 'falling apart' and because the disease was so riddled with irregularity, our conversations would sometimes linger on the possibility of her never recovering from the MS. There were numerous 'miracle cures' in the works. Sometimes we found them in magazine articles or newspapers, but more regularly they were on the internet, which meant that the truth of the testimonials and the evidence supporting the claims was always suspect.

Once, we found a 'cure' in a magazine that boasted sensational results, I called the number provided, but when I began to ask questions, the results were based on a very small test group, the medicine was not FDA approved and would only be available for widespread use in the next two years. I tried to have them use Jemma as a test sample for the product but they told me they did not have the need for any more 'guinea pigs'.

It seemed that the possibilities of her conquering the disease were slowly disappearing as her health worsened and the steroids failed to overcome even the most basic symptoms.

- If it gets any worse - She said - I don't think I can carry on.

- What do you mean, Angel?

- Just that I'm not prepared to struggle any more than I have to. I can put up with a lot, but the idea of becoming totally immobile is enough to make me want to kill myself.

I looked at her, I studied her face and I pondered a reply. I knew this was a turning point for her, and so my answer would determine where our relationship would go from here - whether I could be fully integrated into her decisions, her state of mind, her future; or whether I would be excluded.

- Okay - I replied, at last - I get it. I mean, I understand. But we can still try to look for ways to make it better, right?

- Yes. I'm not giving up, yet. I just want to be very clear on this. I have thought about it long and hard and there is no way I want to be here if I become a burden to you or to myself. I feel like I'm already too much to deal with, so if it looks like I'm not going to be able to manage my own life, then I don't want to live.

How Angels Die - A Confession

She was talking about the possibility of a total blackout, when all the rooms in her body went dark and she could no longer function alone, completely reliant upon others for her survival. She continued

- Life doesn't mean enough to me for me to struggle anymore than necessary. I think about this all the time; already I'm in a situation that makes it hard for me to want to be here. I don't think that I'm important enough to hang around if I'm miserable.

- Are you miserable, Angel?

- Sometimes. Sometimes, yes I am. It's so difficult to do so many things that I feel like a waste of space, and the more I think about it, the more I realize how unimportant I am to the big picture; we are all just ants anyway, so if I'm not here, it won't make any difference and at least I will have been released from this, this prison.

- It will make a difference to me - I said - But I know what you are saying and I'm the last one to judge you for a point of view I hold myself. I understand. I do. Just so long as you keep fighting as hard as you can for as long as you can.

There. We had said it. We agreed. I understood. A silent pact had been made. For Jemma, it was just the comfort of knowing that I would be a support, not a hindrance; this made all the difference for her. She knew she was free to talk to me about it at anytime, and over the next few weeks, actually, for the rest of her life, this type of conversation became a daily ritual for us.

Often, she would show me things she had researched on the internet that related to suicide. Either she would have found stories of people who tried to kill themselves, or she might have seen a video clip of someone actually doing it. There was a blog from one person who had tried and failed - they had placed a plastic bag over their head, securing it around their neck, after which they tied their hands behind their back in the hope of preventing themselves from relenting and undoing the ties around their neck; the intention was suffocation, which would lead to a moment of panic and then death. The outcome was peculiar. Reportedly, they woke up hours later with the bags and the ties all neatly folded in the corner of the room; they had survived. Other blogs discussed various alternative methods of suicide that all seemed agonizing at worst or erratic at best. At one point Jemma even said

- I had a friend at school whose father committed suicide. He waited until the middle of night and drove his car full speed into the wall of the mall. He died instantly.

- You can't do it that way - I commented.

- Why not?

- Because cars today are far safer and you might survive, which would be a fate worse than death, don't you think?

- Yes it would - She agreed - but if I didn't wear a seat belt then the airbags wouldn't go off and it might work.

- Might? - I questioned - Might work?

- You're right - She concluded - It's not full proof enough.

The basic conclusion of all of the searching, the stories, the evidence and the theories was that the human instinct to survive is very powerful and sometimes overwhelming. To kill oneself is no easy task unless you want to suffer horribly in the process.

Despite the facts that stared her in the face, despite knowing how difficult it was to succeed in a suicide, Jemma continued to make it very clear to me on many occasions that she had no desire to live any longer than necessary, especially if she became what she called "a burden."

Rather than say anything to discourage her, which would only serve to distance her from me, I said only those things that I felt would bring comfort. I felt that I was in no position to judge her words or her actions in this and despite my reservations I had basically supported her argument with my own views on suicide. After all, the 37 on my left bicep was a constant reminder of my fickle words that now came back to haunt me.

If I had known how deeply these opinions would have affected me in the end, I doubt I would have raised them in the first place, but now that they were out in the open I felt trapped into upholding them no matter how right or wrong that view may be. I feared being viewed as a hypocrite in her eyes, and if I am totally honest I could, on a logical level, completely understand her position and her desire for an outcome that reduced or eliminated her suffering.

Her love towards me was unconditional and I repaid that love by supporting her decision whatever it might be. No matter how much I might want to help her get well or care for her when things got too much, there was a part of me, (I do not know if 'compassionate' is the word I should use to describe that part of me), but there was a part of me that wanted her to be happy whatever that cost might be. I knew that most people would object or discourage her, and so I made it my business to let her talk it through, to help her come to terms with her words and thoughts; to be there in whatever capacity she might need me.

I am not religious, neither was Jemma, so we were not hindered by the fear of retribution from above. Jemma was logical and practical. So am I. Our thoughts were, initially, totally hypothetical and geared towards a worst case scenario which we hoped would never come to fruition.

As the illness took an even more terrifying hold on her and as the reality of total paralysis became clear, these discussions naturally turned to the cold hard facts that stared us in the face - she would eventually become "a vegetable", "a burden" to herself and to others, helpless yet completely aware. It was an untenable position for her to even contemplate.

Because of this, and because of her views towards death becoming more and more unemotional, we were confronted by the reality of her death everyday for the last six months of her life and in that time I had to say goodbye more than once.

18

She took fifty-eight sleeping pills the first time. I was leaving for Seattle on a weekend work trip which gave her the time to complete her wish, and it gave me an alibi.

Our goodbye was, for want of a better word, surreal.

She sat at the dining table and swallowed the pills very quickly, washing them down with whisky from a small bottle I had bought at the liquor store the day before. I was sitting on the chair diagonally across from her, my mind vacant, my eyes observing. It was sometime after 10PM on a Friday night at the end of June.

Once she became drowsy, I helped her slowly walk down the corridor to her bedroom and then I lifted her onto the bed and pulled the covers over her. Neither of us said a word. I lay in bed next to her for the rest of the night, watching her sleep, watching her breath, watching the clock as the minutes passed evermore slowly.

How Angels Die - A Confession

I was in a state of limbo and I had suspended my belief system so that I could allow her to perform this 'ritual'; I was exhausted from trying to process such a monumental decision, trying to accept such a monumental state of events.

My eyes were heavy from being physically tired, my heart was null and void from the emotional consequences of these actions and agreements. I was not sure if I was betraying myself for allowing her to do it, or whether I was betraying her with my silent acceptance of her wishes.

We had discussed the process numerous times, and, as with everything relating to this, Jemma wanted it to be done with as little fuss as possible. She was deteriorating at an unacceptable speed and she verbalized her situation this way:

- I can feel my body failing me every day. I know that, sooner than I can imagine, I will be immobile, my arms and my hands will get weak and I won't be able to do anything for myself but I will be aware, my mind will still be active. It's not as if I have any responsibilities here, I have no children and I'm not that close with my family. Life is no longer fun for me... I'm stuck in this apartment day and night and I can hardly bear to look at myself anymore. I'm not used to what I see and it upsets me to know that this is the best it will be, it will only get worse from here. I'm sorry, Monkey, I don't mean to be heartless but I think you understand what I'm saying when I say I have no real reason to be here, no reason to live with this situation, nothing to make me stay. I want to end it now, before I get to the point where I can't do it on my own. That would be the worst for me, much worse than death.

These words meandered through my mind as I lay next to her on that Friday night, fighting off my exhaustion, controlling my emotions. I thought about the state of her mind as she took the pills, the disconnection she must have felt to be able to take her own life.

I had often thought of or talked about suicide as a possibility, but it was just a passing whim in a moment of frustration that did not go to the depths of the act, the motions it required to be able to accept death, the finality of it all, knowing that one particular action would end everything - one moment you exist and the next you do not. Added to that was the uncertainty that followed, the complete lack of knowledge we have of the afterlife, if there even is one.

When it comes to life after death, I have my ideas, I have my theories, I have my fears, but when it comes to the death of one you love, all of these are discarded in the hope that this person will return, even if it is just for a moment, so you can experience them again, for one last time.

The deeper my thoughts became, the less I was able to comprehend and the more my eyes welled up with tears as I imagined trying to carry on without Jemma. It was a reality that I could not begin to truly contemplate despite being confronted with it in the most inexplicable way.

I stirred myself very early that Saturday morning, after having watched her throughout the night in a kind of mental haze. I left the apartment at 5:30AM to go to the gym before I went home, packed my bags and flew out to Seattle. We had agreed that I should stick to my schedule in order that there was nothing that might implicate me in her decision to commit suicide - I was therefore left with little choice but to try to do what I normally would in the most mundane way possible.

When I got up she was breathing almost too lightly for it to be discernible, she was lying on her back, her eyes closed, her body motionless. She seemed to be at peace and so when I left her, I left without thinking that she would really die, without having completed the thoughts and the actions as I probably should have.

Perhaps I could not handle the truth of the situation, perhaps I was in denial. I certainly was not thinking clearly or rationally. As I walked away from her in the cold morning light, my tears were plentiful, if full of doubt that this performance was for real. I was empty of recognition for what we were doing, of the finality of the last few hours.

How Angels Die - A Confession

When I got to the gym and was in the presence of others I managed to act as if everything was the same as always, I suppressed my tears, I averted my eyes from anyone I might recognize. I moved as if I was a ghost. I was well aware that I could not give the game away, for her sake, despite my incredulity.

While I was at home packing my bags I overcame moments of sadness by pretending it was just my over-active imagination getting the better of me. I told myself that I could not be defeated now, I had to be strong in these terrible hours of uncertainty. Something inside me was switched off; it was as if I was surviving with my senses dulled - this was a necessary part of the equation if I was going to pull through for Jemma.

As I got to the boarding gate at LAX in the late afternoon to fly out, my phone rang.

The screen read: Angel.

I hesitated before picking up the phone, afraid of what I might hear, terrified that she had succeeded, hopeful that she had failed. I did not know who would be at the other end of the line as I accepted the call.

It was Jemma, she had woken up. I was struck by conflicting emotions in the same instant, I was relieved for myself, yet momentarily upset for her. The pills had not worked. She was distraught with confusion and irritation at surviving, I felt useless as I tried to calm her down. What should she do? What went wrong? I questioned whether I should even go to Seattle but she told me to get on the plane, she assured me she would be alright, she did not want me to come back to look after her.

When I eventually landed in Seattle after a short flight that seemed to last an eternity I very nearly returned to LA before I left the airport. I called her as we touched down, I told her how conflicted I felt, I offered to come back, to be with her, to help her get over it, but she insisted that she wanted to be alone; it was her tone of determination that made me stay in Seattle, nothing else.

Over the next day we spoke regularly.

- I think I want to try to slit my wrists - She said - I have a sharp knife here.

- No, Angel. No - I demanded - What happens if you make a mistake and only hurt yourself, what if you end up lying there for hours in agony? Please, don't do anything right now. I'll be back soon and we can work out what to do then.

- Okay - She acquiesced - But I just feel so frustrated, lying here on the sofa. I feel like I want to do something.

- I'm so sorry, Angel - I replied - I really am, but if you're going to do this, it has to be full proof, we cannot leave this job half done and I cannot deal with you doing it with a knife, it's too uncertain.

She was silent for a moment and then she agreed.

- You're right - She said - I don't think I could do it properly with a knife, it scares me to even think about it.

I had discouraged her because I felt she might not be strong enough mentally or physically to complete the task and I could not imagine her having to cope with the aftermath of another failed attempt. I did not discourage her for any other reason. I understood her frustration and I felt her anguish and fear. I encouraged her to have Christina visit, to break the monotony, but I still worried that she might try to do something, so my trip to Seattle was extremely unsettling, and the trip home came all too slowly.

I got to her apartment as quickly as I could on the Sunday evening and I did everything I could to be a pillar of strength for her in her time of need, fear and angst. At my behest, she had refrained from trying anything else and so I felt a responsibility now for all her suffering. No matter what I said to try to appease her anguish I did not feel convincing, despite my relief at still having her to hold close to me.

And then she said, quite simply

- I want to do it with a gun.

How Angels Die - A Confession

She was in my arms, we were on the sofa, she had stopped crying, we were in a state of limbo, that place where the storm has quieted down but there is a sense of foreboding in the air. As she said it, I felt her body strengthen with resolve while my body became weak with the implications of what she meant. I tried not to show a reaction.

- Okay - I uttered - Why?

- Because that is the only certain way to die. Every other way can fail. If I don't succeed in this soon I'll have to ask you to do it for me later and as much as I know you'll do anything for me, that would not be fair.

- It can fail with a gun, Angel. It can leave you maimed for life. It is a brutal and vicious method to choose.

- I know. And it worries me to do it that way too, but I can no longer live like this and I can't afford to fail again. Time is running out. I want to get a gun and I want to finish this...

She drifted off. And yet again, I played along; out of pure love I allowed myself to go along with her wishes, for her sake, for her peace of mind, for her dignity. I did not like it one little bit, I felt completely nauseous, I did not want her to have to use a gun, I did not want to be a part of it; but I did not want to let her down, I did not want her to suffer anymore, I did not want her to doubt how unconditional my love was.

- And how will I explain this? - I asked, in a moment of selfishness.

- You can say I got it for my own protection for when you are away. Now that I can't defend myself against an intruder, I need a gun. And, that's the truth anyway. I am scared when I'm alone.

She had already thought about it and she had already decided. I was left with no choice. As the decision sunk in, as it became clear that I would have to be involved in this and I would be further embroiled in something so confusing for my heart and my head, I was extremely uncomfortable - she had absolutely no knowledge of handguns and I felt that it was the wrong way for her to end her life. Girls do not shoot themselves, I thought. My Angel was too soft, too fragile, too elegant to die that way. But again, I was aware that my dissension would only serve to alienate me from her life and so I allowed myself to believe that she was getting the gun for her own protection when I was traveling, a gun that she would hopefully never have to use. There was no other way for me to justify her owning a weapon that could do so much harm.

She went through the rigamarole of choosing, buying and legally obtaining a handgun, small enough for her to control in her weakened state, yet powerful enough to do the trick should she actually decide to perform this task.

How Angels Die - A Confession

One cloudy weekday afternoon, I carried her to my car and we drove to the gun shop on Sunset near Doheny. Once we had parked, I carried her to the elevator and into the store as she was too weak to walk; she quickly chose and paid for the gun and took the required test booklet home to study. A day later we went back. I carried her to and from the car, and to and from the store - she passed the test, which meant the gun would be hers in ten days.

- Will you show me how to use it? - She asked - And also, what do I need to do to make sure I don't harm anyone else?

Even in her darkest hour, Jemma was still concerned about others, about making sure she did not disrupt anyone else's life while she ended hers. In this, as in all things, she disarmed me.

Once we arrived at the apartment and I had settled her comfortably in one of the chairs by the dining table, I went through all the necessary safety regulations and procedures with her, the things she had not quite grasped at the gun shop. It was disconcerting having to explain the workings of a firearm, supposing that its sole purpose would be to end a life, her life.

- I should put the gun in my mouth when I do it, shouldn't I?

How Angels Die - A Confession

We had seen a video of someone who had shot themselves through the roof of the mouth and the victim seemed to die instantly.

- Yes - I replied - But if you look at that video you will see he pushed the gun to the roof of the mouth, pointing at his brain, and he held it very firmly. There is a strong kick when the trigger is pulled.

It completely sickened me to say these words, it shattered me emotionally to think that I was having to talk to My Angel about this as if we were two people discussing somebody else. I was aware that I could not show any sadness towards her in these moments, she would not be grateful to me for making it any more difficult than it already was.

She went over everything again - where to lie on the bed, where to place the pillows to stop any collateral damage, how to hold the gun, what to expect when she pulled the trigger - until she seemed to understand clearly what was required of her to make this attempt successful.

Once we had gone over everything about the gun, she asked me to put it in her bedside table with the cartridges next to it, and then she wanted to watch television.

I helped her from the dining chair to the sofa, I lay her down and put her legs over my lap as I sat near her. With my eyes on the screen I slowly processed that she had never fired a gun before, she had never even held one that was loaded. A feeling of total misunderstanding washed over me as I thought about her pulling the trigger for the first time. It would be the last voluntary movement she ever made. My whole being slumped as I thought about the disconnection of her having to do something she had never done before in order that she could escape the torment she was experiencing now.

The irony was not lost on me, the first time she would do something being the last thing she ever did. More than that, I was fearful she would not perform her task successfully as she was a novice with firearms. The thought rested for a moment, and then wrestled with me. The concern did not leave me. I said nothing, I watched the screen, I tried to put the thought out of my head, I had to be present for her.

I did not know how much longer I would have her.

19

A week or so later she said

- I want to do it on Friday afternoon.

- Okay, Angel.

There was nothing else I could say.

I went to the bedside table and took out the gun. I looked it over and then handed it to her. She loaded the magazine with ten cartridges as I watched. Then, I checked the safety catch and replaced the gun in the drawer.

On the Friday, I arranged to see an afternoon movie with a friend of mine who was visiting from England.

Before I left Jemma's apartment I helped her stand up. We stood face to face, my hands in her long brown hair and her head against my chest. I could not quite believe that she could be gone forever in the next few minutes. The finality of this decision seemed to come from a place that I could not fathom, a place that did not exist in our world. She was My Angel. She would always be My Angel. Nothing could take that away from me, could it?

We stood there for a while nervously holding on to each other before I kissed her slowly and repeatedly on the forehead and then I looked into her eyes, confused as to how I should let go, how to walk away. In the end, she was the one to speak, and she spoke calmly, it seemed that she was resigned to her fate, but she said nothing directly.

- I hope everything works out for you. I hope you are happy. Please try to be happy. I love you so very much.

For a moment or two I just looked into her eyes. I tried to crack a smile, but instead, tears streamed down my face, just as they do now when I write these words. She looked at me and then began to kiss my tears away ever so softly. I was now holding her shoulders, preparing to walk away, but unable to let go for the final time. I stood there, hoping to stall the inevitable. I pulled her back in close to me, tears still falling, my voice weak.

- I love you, Angel. And I always will. Always.

It took every piece of me to finally break away from her. It broke every piece of my heart to turn my back on her, to open the door and then close it, to step outside and continue moving. I walked away in the pouring rain and when I turned back to look at her window, she had the blind pulled back and she was waving her farewell, a small, timid wave, like a child wishing that their parent would not leave them to fend for themselves. She was watching me, saying goodbye to me, letting me know that this was it, her wish was to be gone despite the love we held for one another, perhaps thanks to that love, perhaps she knew she was so loved that she felt it was all she needed to be able to leave. I had to allow her that freedom, as much as my wish would have been very different if I had been allowed just one wish.

I do not remember the movie or the actors. I sat there, numb to the world as I wondered if she had pulled the trigger now... now... now...

My mind swirled back to the week before when she had asked how to do it. I suppose I was hoping she would never decide to - yet, as much as it seemed unnatural to me at the time, it was preferable that she knew what to do and succeeded rather than making a failed attempt that could leave her even worse off.

I had watched her load the gun, I had put the safety on. Should I have done this? Probably not, but my thoughts these days were far from acceptable, they were simply practical; Jemma's wishes became more important than my desires.

We had discussed where she should lie, how to place the pillows, exactly where the end of the barrel should go in her mouth, at which point she should let the safety off and only then should she place her finger on the trigger. I warned her of the recoil that might effect the location of entry and the speed of death. I tried to make something so vicious and so wrong seem simple and clean in order that she might be able to complete the task with confidence. Now, if this had to be the way, I just hoped that it would be quick and painless.

No matter how hard I tried to think positively about something so damaging, I kept drifting back to the possibility that something might go wrong and she might be lying there alone, helpless and in agony...

As my friend and I walked out of the movie, my phone rang. I looked at the screen:

Angel

I answered the call without hesitation.

- It won't work - She said - I tried three times. I counted to ten and I tried to pull the trigger but I think it's jammed.

My body collapsed inside itself. I was overwhelmed with the information. I was distraught and pained, for me, for her.

- Are you okay? - I asked.

- I don't know, I don't know...

How Angels Die - A Confession

- I'll be there in ten minutes.

I turned to my friend.

- I have to go. Sorry - I spurted.

I stayed on the phone with Jemma as I ran to my car and drove back to the apartment, I was shaking, but I did my best to calm myself so that I could be strong for her. I was selfishly relieved that it had not worked, our goodbye had seemed wrong, not the farewell I had imagined, if I had even imagined a farewell at all.

When I arrived back at her apartment I held her happily in my arms as the tears and anguish fell quietly and gently from her saddened blue eyes and her jaded, broken heart.

We were together again and that was all that mattered at that moment - I tried not to think about her lying on the bed a few moments before, alone, a pillow behind her head, the cold steel barrel of a gun jammed into her mouth as she decided that now was the time to let everything go. I tried not to imagine her as she slowly yet deliberately counted to ten and finally applied pressure to the slim trigger, squeezing gently - terrified, nervous, expectant for the shocking explosion that would ricochet through her entire being. That moment of finality evading her and being replaced by a palpable sense of fear that she had survived and had to endure yet another useless day.

How Angels Die - A Confession

How had she decided that today was the day? How had she managed to find the courage to put the gun in her mouth? How had she built up the mental and physical strength to actually pull at the trigger? And how must she feel now as she softly wept tears of frustration, confusion and agonizing relief?

I tried to think only of the fact that she was back in my arms, her body was warm and we would spend another day together. That, for me at least, would be a day of relative happiness, because I would see her again. But it was hard to be selfish when I knew that all she really wanted was to be gone. It broke my heart to have to live with this dilemma, to have to assist in the final demise of a person that I loved so strongly, but if I loved her unconditionally, then that love allowed me no choice.

- I don't think I can do it with a gun, it's too brutal. Too immediate. I want to try with pills again - She finally said.

- Alright, Angel. Whatever you want.

I felt a huge sense of relief that she was not going to use a bullet to end her life and I acquiesced as a way of keeping her close to me. She was determined and desperate, that I knew.

Jemma had a sense that she was on a time limit and she had to do something while she could. She was convinced that sooner rather than later her body would simply shut down completely and she would be unable to carry out her final wish, she would be too weak to even hold the gun.

Who was I to stop her or interfere or hinder her? What did I know of her struggle, the mental anguish she endured throughout the day, the emptiness she must have felt, the loneliness and frustration in the hours when I was not there? I could not judge. I could not prevent her from achieving that wish. It was not my choice, or my place to do anything other than love her in her hour of need. I was left with no option if I wanted to remain a part of her life. I could only hope that something, one thing, the smallest thing might change, and that event, that moment would derail this process that she had set in motion.

I lived with these thoughts day in and day out. These thoughts ate me up inside, I was in an untenable position that only left me with loss.

If I refused to help her, I would lose her, she would not be able to express herself with me which would mean separation on some level and she would therefore be left alone to conclude the final chapter of her life; I loved her too much to leave her to fend for herself when she needed me.

If I allowed her to end her life, if I continued in my silent assistance, then I not only guaranteed losing her, I also created for myself a future that would never let me be free of that loss and the manner in which it occurred.

This terrible dichotomy, this feeling of guilt for wanting her to achieve her goals aligned with this fear of losing her forced me into a situation where I had to discount my own emotions in order to be able to assist her in understanding hers. As much as I wanted to express myself and allow myself the luxury of contemplation, I was all too aware that weakness was not an option for me should I consider my love to be unconditional, which I did.

Confronted with these choices, I felt that her will to die was unwavering and this left me as the unwilling, yet complicit participant in her deadly plans.

Over the next six weeks she collected more sleeping pills - she was prescribed thirty from her doctor and she gathered up others from websites that would send the medication in from Canada. One evening when I came into the apartment, she said to me

- I called my doctor and told her that I had accidentally dropped my pills down the toilet, she's sent in a prescription for thirty more; will you go and pick it up for me?

- Yes, Angel. I'll go now.

I did not question her, I did not pry, I simply went to Rite Aid on Sunset Boulevard as I always did when she needed prescriptions; it had been months since she could do these things for herself. I had stood in the line countless times before to pick up medication. It was a grim task that only served to remind me that her life was unbearable.

My soul emptied out when I thought about what she was going through, how despondent she must feel, how solitary the decision she was making had to be. As I walked through the parking lot with the paper bag in my hand, I hoped that this time it would all work out the way she had planned. It might not have been the way she would have chosen, but she had few options with this decision and this was the most painless way to end her life. There had been many occasions over the past year when she had said to me and to others

- I wish I could just go to sleep and never wake up.

I think this is the way that most of us would wish for, given the choice, but unfortunately, we are not given the choice and death seems to be either a sudden, tragic event, or a slow, lingering episode we would all rather be spared; which one will befall us we never know until it is too late. In this case, Jemma was trying to turn a slow, lingering episode into a painless and peaceful finale, one that would enable her to avoid the emotional trauma and physical demise that her body was preparing for her. I, for my part, was playing the role that I would not have chosen. Yet, if I professed to love her as I did, this was the only role my love would allow. It was a painful role indeed.

How Angels Die - A Confession

When I arrived back at her apartment with the pills, she said quietly

- I want to do it on Saturday morning. I have enough pills now.

I hid my sadness, my shock, my devastation; I just nodded my head in agreement, I kept my eyes down and sat next to her on the sofa. I entwined her fingers in mine and tilted my head towards hers until the side of our heads were touching.

Her words had been absent of any feeling, any emotion. The decision was now practical. I realized - for her, all emotion had to be discounted if she was to carry this through. As I think back, I remember her attitude becoming one of function; life was empty now, she had my love which was her one joy, but she had no hope.

Without hope, we have nothing to live for.

20

Hope is the one thing that keeps humans alive, it is the intangible product of life that allows us to suffer interminably without giving up - Jemma had lost all hope.

The medication no longer served its purpose, it only served up confusion - should she fight on because she could move a little, should she give up despite the fact that she was not in constant pain? It had come to the point where her instinct to survive had been ripped from her and now she only saw the futility in life.

If our survival instinct is to be based on anything, I would offer up a choice of three - fear, ego and hope - Jemma was left with none of these. This is not to say she was depressed - I know that she felt enormous sadness and she probably had moments of depressive thinking, but above all, Jemma was a positive person who never projected her worries onto others.

Despite our closeness she did not dwell on the negative parts of our existence, she mentioned her feelings in passing more than she analyzed them, and she seemed to be comfortable with the fact that I understood her enough to know that once a subject had been broached and dealt with, then it was not something she generally delved into again.

Naturally, as a communicative and caring couple, we would talk often of the way she felt, of the possibilities or impossibilities before us, but there was a limit to how much we hashed over the same things. These discussions always ended with her saying

- I don't want to be sad. I'm so lucky in so many ways. I have you. I love you.

And that was that - we would then move on to our evening of watching TV on the sofa, ordering club sandwiches on white bread from Yummy Home Delivery, eating the most terrible desserts because it did not matter anymore, and drinking soda pops or sugar filled drinks because they tasted so damn good. By this stage I had given up all hope of trying to get Jemma to change her diet. It had been a difficult battle for me to continue with when I knew she was fighting so much in the first place, and so now I resigned myself to making the most of the moments we were together. I would lie with my head on her lap and she would gently massage my face until I became drowsy from her tenderness, I was spoilt by her love, I loved it and I took full advantage of it in the most loving way possible. I knew that it was a privilege to be so adored by her and I never took that for granted.

How Angels Die - A Confession

Once in a while, reality hit us in the face when she suddenly needed to go to the bathroom without warning and she would not be able to get up off the sofa. I would carry her there without comment and would help her if she wanted. Usually she wanted to be left alone. I would wait until she called me...

- Monkey?

- Yes, My Angel... Coming.

Multiple Sclerosis is a vicious disease, not least because it leaves the victim totally aware of the debilitation. If it takes a hold before one is thirty, then the onset is more rapid. After forty, it is generally a slower process that might take two or more decades to completely shatter a life. For Jemma, it took less than six years to be beyond unacceptable - the process was merciless and unpredictable - it would offer up hope for a few days and then it would crush all hope in an instant. The disease was constantly there despite everything seemingly being normal. Even with the medical concoctions of powerful steroids there was no knowing what the next few hours would bring. Nothing could be planned because most functions of the body became uncontrollable, and of course, the more one worried about it the worse these issues became.

We had talked long and hard about 'positive reinforcement', even 'the power of the subconscious', or 'mind over matter' and 'the need to overcome'; yet these thoughts and these talks did not have the desired effect and when a relapse occurred it simply negated all positive thinking because she had been making an effort to think positively and it was not working. What was the point?

Jemma decided everything was pointless - she had no dependents. She was in more regular contact with her Christina, but was not that emotionally attached, and although she came to visit regularly with Anthony in the last few months of Jemma's life, which Jemma enjoyed now that she was housebound, I know it was hard for her to forget the past. Her mother lived in Denver and Jemma rarely saw her or her other sister, Katie. Jemma had a few friends, but nobody that she felt responsible for; she knew that I fully understood and respected her view on death. And so, she decided that there was nothing to live for, no point holding on now, no reason to struggle through the days when it would make no difference anyway.

Added to all of this was the physical change in her body, which was giving up on her as well, leaving her with the possibility of becoming immobile, and this was too much for her to contemplate. She had made her decision and now she was carrying it out.

There were a couple of occasions, towards the end of her life, when she asked me

- Why do you keep coming to see me? Why do you stay here with me? Isn't it depressing for you?

How Angels Die - A Confession

She had become so despondent inside her heart that she could not even understand why I would want to be around her anymore. It completely and utterly shattered me to hear those words. I struggled to maintain my composure as I replied

- Because I love you, Angel. Because you're a special and sweet person, and I love being with you. We always have fun and I miss you when I'm not with you.

- But you should be enjoying yourself, you should be with people who can do things with you. You should be able to find love elsewhere...

She drifted off, but I could not leave those words hanging in the air. I knew what she was saying. I had not been perfect, of that I was all too aware, but I also knew that I did not want to be apart from Jemma. I knew I would be with her for as long as I could be, for as long as life would allow. And so, when she spoke of me being with other people in the roundabout way that she did, I was ready to respond, ready to quash her doubts, or fears.

- I want to be with you. I don't want to be anywhere else. Please know that, and please try to understand how important you are to me, how much I care for you and how much I enjoy being with you.

How Angels Die - A Confession

She would just look at me, confused that I would value our time together when it seemed so repetitive to her. She was saddened we had "come to this."

I could see the pain in her eyes as she looked at me sometimes while I did all of the little mundane tasks she could no longer perform. It gave me pleasure to help her, to be with her, to enjoy her company, to spend our evenings together, to go to sleep next to her every night, to wake up with her every morning.

Although she was feeling immense sadness, she would never transfer it onto me. We always talked happily and I would always give her kisses whenever we were near each other. She would smile and laugh often; her greeting as I walked in the door was always full of joy and happiness.

She was a truly beautiful person, someone who was kind to everyone she met and who only wanted life to be simple and easy. Now, her life was not simple or easy, it was complicated and confusing, it had taken her to a place where she no longer saw the value of her existence, and she could not see why I would spend time with her.

For me, time with her was, and always had been, something I looked forward to in every way. In some ways, I sensed it was more precious now than ever before.

As I mentioned earlier, she had often said in the last few months that she wished she would go to sleep and never wake up - I never felt offended by this. I knew that she loved me dearly, deeply and purely; we had been together for nearly seven years and I had watched her slowly disintegrate before my eyes. I had witnessed her health decline until it became intolerable, especially in the last two years. Her mind still functioned perfectly, yet her body would no longer respond. Her level of frustration must have been unimaginable to you or I.

As a lively, attractive and charismatic girl who was used to compliments and positive attention, it must have been incredibly difficult to comprehend this new existence which required loss of pride, some shame, and worst of all, pity.

21

Some doctors believe that Multiple Sclerosis is a defective gene that lies dormant in the body waiting to be triggered by a traumatic event which then kick starts the disease.

In essence, MS strips away the protective layer of the nerves, sometimes quickly, sometimes sparodically, sometimes very slowly. This then exposes the nerves which consequently confuses the message that the brain gives to the body, and ultimately the information either travels incorrectly, or not at all.

MS is a rampant disease, yet it seems to be different for every person that is victim to it. For some it is painful, for others, not at all. For some it affects the legs, for others the hands. Sometimes the disease hits and remains constant, at other times it hits and then retreats. Often, the MS mercilessly strikes and then continues to attack until death. No two patients have the same story.

Multiple Sclerosis is also notoriously difficult to diagnose accurately - it resembles other diseases and, as the symptoms are different in most cases, there are always other possibilities. During Jemma's last few weeks, we had to endure this cruelty.

She had been assigned to a new doctor for her home care who had said, almost immediately

- I don't think you have MS.

This was a ray of hope that we could never have imagined only a day before. If it was not MS, then that would explain why the steroids were not working as effectively as they should. It would mean that she could have different medication to treat a different disease; this could mean a new lease of life - literally. There would be no more talk of suicide, no more suicide attempts, no more fear of losing her, just a cure and a process, a series of medical procedures to follow in order to correct the wrongs of the past few years. This could be a new beginning for her, for us.

The doctor asked if Jemma would be prepared to undergo some tests to eliminate the possibility of MS. Jemma asked me if I would be able to help her get to the appointments. The answer to each question was a resounding yes.

With this glimmer of hope, Jemma readied herself for some good news, and she prepared herself before each set of impending visits. I would make sure to have the day free so I could be with her the whole time.

How Angels Die - A Confession

In the morning, we would wake up and shower, I would help her dress and sit with her while she put on her make up. We would have a small breakfast and then I would carry her to the car, or, if it was a good day I would be her walking stick.

We would drive to the hospitals or medical facilities and Jemma would undergo a series of tests, blood samples, physical examinations or MRI's. Changing out of her clothes and into the robes was an ordeal in itself. On top of this were the car journeys that she had to endure, as well as the wheelchair rides through the corridors where she felt so self-conscious. The medical tests were a physical and an emotional strain, but it was worth it because it might lead to new possibilities - there might be hope for a cure, or at the very least, a reprieve.

After a month of backwards and forwards, of possibilities and renewed energy, we went to meet with the doctor in charge of the testing procedures - she sat us in a small room and she opened her files. She looked at us, we were holding hands as usual, and she asked Jemma if she wanted to be alone, or if she wanted me in the room.

- I would like him to stay - She replied.

The doctor paused for a moment. Then she looked directly at Jemma. She hesitated.

- I'm afraid that it is definitely MS you have. There is no other explanation.

Jemma's hand went limp in mine. She looked down, and tears welled up in her eyes. I looked across at Jemma, helpless, my heart breaking for her; for me.

After a moment, the doctor asked Jemma about the steroids she was taking and the effect they were having. She confirmed the medication Jemma was taking was the best available. She mentioned physical therapy and other forms of assistance; she asked Jemma if there was anything she needed to know and she gave Jemma her contact information.

I held Jemma's hand the whole time and squeezed it gently. I could sense the defeat, and I knew that she had been dealt the final blow. The doctor then left us alone in the room and as the door closed Jemma began to cry. So did I.

- Why me? - She finally sobbed - I don't understand why I have this. Why I'm defective and Christina isn't? If it's genetic, then why am I the only one who has it?

I held her, wrapped in my arms, her head in my chest, her tears warm on my shirt. I was at a loss for an explanation; there was no explanation.

- I don't know, Angel - I replied - It's not fair. That much I do know. And I hate that you're going through this.

How Angels Die - A Confession

She was silent for a little while, her sobbing slowed down and she finally moved her head from my chest to my shoulder.

- Not for much longer - She said - I won't be going through this for much longer.

Despite her previous attempts at suicide, she had not lost her positivity or her warm demeanor. Those attempts had been her way of stopping the needless anguish of a life that held no hope, of making sure she did not become an object that could not function. In those dark days there was no cure, no way out. Yet those attempts at suicide had failed. Was there a reason for the failure? And then, out of nowhere she had been offered a possibility and the chance to maybe correct the misalignment in her system, a slither of light.

She was shattered by what just happened - a ray of possibility followed by a devastating lightning strike - this disappointment was unendurable. There was no hope left.

There was no point taking steroids that did not work, there were no other steroids to take; there was no reason to feel ill anymore in the hope that she might one day recover. She knew she would never get better and would eventually end up immobile, a 'burden.'

MS had physically, emotionally and spiritually taken the life out of My Angel. Now, it was just a matter of how and when her end would come.

22

My brother, Gabriel, was three years younger than me, and much better looking. He had high round cheekbones, full lips and big blue eyes, a thick head of hair, beautiful skin.

But, he was terminally ill. At the age of four he was diagnosed with Batten's; a degenerative disease that is deadly. Before it kills, it maims and paralyses, disables and destroys.

As a small boy I had to watch my younger brother, an even smaller boy, endure epileptic seizures that led to spasticity, to vegetation, to blindness. The stages were heartless.

Initially, he went to school in an ambulance until he could no longer walk; this was before he went blind. In the end, he lay helpless in bed as his undeveloped mind lay dormant and his ailing body disintegrated.

We fed him with liquids that went from a plastic cup through a tube into his nose and down into his stomach. His muscles disappeared and he became stick thin. My mother wrapped sheepskin around his knees and elbows to stop his skin from chaffing. We had nurses for him periodically and whenever we went on vacation I would accompany my parents and Gabriel to a hospital for the terminally ill. We lay him on duvets and pillows in the trunk of our family car and I would keep an eye on him as we drove.

When we arrived we would carry his dead weight to the wheelchair and we would wheel him to his designated bed. What I saw there possibly shaped what I am now. There were soulless wards along covered walkways. In those wards were beds that held small, deformed, erratic, aimless, vacant children. They were all, without exception, helpless. They were all pale and frail. They were all going to die before I finished school.

On the one hand, seeing those things at a young age gave me compassion. I never looked at anyone with a disability as if they were different. I knew they had a family, loved ones, even friends, dreams and beliefs.

I was exposed to nature's cruelty and it influenced my perspective on everything. I was confronted with possibilities and impossibilities when I was not old enough to comprehend anything differently. I knew that if fate had dealt me a slightly different hand it could have been me in the back of the car, surrounded by soft padding, lying there, in a world that nobody could enter and nobody could fully understand.

How Angels Die - A Confession

I grew up with a brutal and incomprehensible reality. It made me sensitive to the needs of others.

On the other hand, these unavoidable miscarriages of justice gave me cause to question good and evil, right and wrong, heaven and hell. I saw no reason for my brother to be struck down by this illness; I saw no reason why my mother should endure these years of care-taking and then the loss of a child; I saw no reason why I had been spared and my brother had been chosen for this pointless purgatory. It was unfair. It was unjust. It was wrong. It showed me that life was harsh and that humans are as insignificant as anything else on the planet.

Gabriel died on December 1st, 1985; the day after his twelfth birthday. I was at boarding school doing my homework in my room when another boy called me to the public phone in the corridor. My father said two words

- He's gone.

That was all he needed to say for me to know my brother was dead, for me to break down and cry, the phone held to my ear, my knees buckling beneath me, my heart stopping. A wasted life snuffed out by an evil illness. An innocent boy selected for unnecessary punishment. Gone. Finished.

I was devastated by his loss, not least because I could not understand it or the point of his life. My mother is the most wonderful, loving, kind, decent, exceptional woman. She rises above others on many levels; she has her faults hidden somewhere, but they are hard to find. For her to have been given this burden made no sense. For her to lose a child, the worst punishment any parent can endure, was wrong.

To deal with deterioration and death at such a young age only served to make me practical, logical and paradoxical. I did not see the goodness in this world, I simply saw the pointless. I know that life does not matter, but while I am here, I am determined it should be easy. I have been dealt the hand of health, wealth and happiness. I refuse to exert myself if I cannot enjoy the act. As far as I am concerned, this life is useless. Death is the ultimate proof for cynical opinions, because in the end we just disappear.

I am certain my views on suicide, my willingness to close off my life in my own way, my desire to control my own demise, my ability to be amused when others are horrified, came from my childhood - from my brother's plight, from the suffering I witnessed and still struggle to understand.

I lost my brother over twenty-five years ago and it still makes no difference to anyone but me and my mother. For everyone else it is just a story. For us, it is a memory, a reflection, an affliction, a tragedy, a bonding, a reason to see beyond what we are taught so that we can deal with what is real.

How Angels Die - A Confession

Mum and I remember the good in Gabriel's life when we talk. We look at it as a positive experience that enables us to handle life in a way that we might not have otherwise known. There is no anger left in either of us over Gabriel's death or the manner of his existence. It is what it is; it was what it was. It will never be anything different.

When I had first met Jemma, I had spoken of Gabriel. When her illness became untenable, I shared my fear of watching another loved one deteriorate and wither away before my eyes. I know she was concerned for me as her body disintegrated. She would mention her fear on occasion; fear she was putting me through the same hell all over again. I told her not to worry. I know she did. Although I tried never to make her feel responsible I know my pain was multiplied two-fold in this situation - a memory and a reality - yet my ability to cope with what she was going through was due to what I had already been through once before.

23

Saturday morning:

She had taken the pills. I had watched almost helplessly as she devoured them and I had waited by her side for her to drift to as near death as I could bear.

As I drove my car away from her apartment to the Sample Sale in downtown L.A. all I could see before me was My Sweet Angel lying in the bed, asleep, looking peaceful and very, very still.

I did not know if she was dead, or whether she was just breathing indiscernibly. I did not know how death should look, or how to tell. I had been too fearful to touch her neck or wrist to feel for a pulse just in case she was only sleeping lightly and I might then scare her into waking up at an early stage of her drowsiness and impede her final wish.

When I had stood at the end of the bed and said my goodbye, I almost could not deal with the fact that she might be dead. It was easier for me to imagine that she was unconscious, that she was still in the process of 'passing on'.

Had she 'gone' by the time I left the apartment? Or had it happened as I drove? Was it happening now? I was numb from the emotional severity of what we were doing. It was, I suppose, better that my emotions were seemingly dulled; this enabled me to deal with this devastating situation in a practical way so I was able to function cohesively in order to 'get the job done' - not for me, but for My Angel.

I arrived at the Sample Sale and stood in the booth. It was full of clothes that were counted as overstock; clothes that I had designed, clothes that were out of season and therefore it was impractical to keep them. These clothes were a cash injection into the business - cash that would otherwise be tied up in a warehouse. The hall was full of people who only communicated on a financial level which made it easier to just be there in a dysfunctional kind of way. I answered their questions with a number and if they bartered with me I simply replied with another number that might appease them.

My mind was elsewhere, in Hollywood, in an apartment, at the foot of a bed in a darkened bedroom where something real was happening that I could no longer reverse. A life was being extinguished out of choice and I would never get the chance to talk to that beautiful person again, I would never hear her voice again, I would never be able to laugh with her, hold her in my arms or speak to her on the phone as I had done every single day for all these years. Everything we had was now in the past, gone, finished, over, an empty history. No matter what, it would all now be a memory that only I would have and as time passed I knew it would be more and more difficult to recall her in my mind's eye. How would I remember the exact feeling of her lips, the touch of her hand or the smell of her skin? And when I could no longer remember it so well, what would that do to me? How empty would I feel? How lost?

I left the booth for a moment, my mind in a haze. My stomach was feeling uncomfortable and my eyes wanted to cry; I felt empty and hollow, the tears caught in my throat. I began to question whether I had done the right thing by allowing her to end her life. I thought about rushing back to the apartment and trying to wake her up, but the thought passed quickly. She would only be upset with me if I did that, and she would only try again another time if I stopped her now.

I snapped out of it. I knew that she would resent me for keeping her alive. It would be an act of pure selfishness on my part. I was well aware that her biggest fear was becoming a "vegetable" reliant upon others for survival, having no dignity left.

That was it, dignity - that was why I was helping her, allowing her to die. It was an inevitable turn of events. She would die one day, somehow, and I would lose her. It was better that it happened on her terms now than in a few years when I would have to be responsible for not allowing her to do what she wished for when she had the opportunity.

24

We had discussed it on many occasions - euthanasia. We were both pragmatic about death; we both had the same feelings. As far as we could see, we were kept alive artificially from the day we were born, we were pumped full of 'artificial preservatives' that quelled the onslaught of so many killer viruses and diseases, whether they be the common cold, flu, tuberculosis, malaria, polio, or even cancer - the human race was living well over twice the expected age of our natural sell-by-date and we had over-populated and destroyed the earth as a result.

Yet, if somebody decided that their life had become, or was about to become unbearable, and they chose death as a viable option, then all of a sudden one was told that euthanasia was illegal because "you can't play God with a human life." It was illogical to Jemma and I that the same view was not held at the other end of the age scale when we were young, with no voice to stop the medical system, yet we were riddled with inoculations - and, beyond the scientific situation we all endure, if human life is sacred, then the form and quality a life holds should be sacred too.

How Angels Die - A Confession

As these thoughts played out in my head during the day, I managed to settle my emotions enough that I could maintain an air of normalcy around other people and I went back to the booth. I was doing the right thing by Jemma. I was enabling her to control her own life and her own death, and that was the greatest gift I could give her right now, or ever.

Although my mind and my heart were understanding I still felt anger towards the situation. I could not quite adjust or accept the fact that I could not be there to ease her into her death. It seemed so wrong that she had to be in a darkened room, solitary, as her body faded away and her spirit left. I wanted to be lying next to her, holding her close, showing her how loved she was as she left this world.

I wanted this to be a positive experience for her, not a frightening one. It should have been a moment when she was surrounded by those who loved her, a time when she could have said her farewells to close friends and family over a few days, when she could have discussed and explained her decision and her situation so that others could acclimatize themselves to the reality of her plight and she could then have had her chance to fare well into a death that would have been accepted and acceptable. Instead, she had to keep all this a secret from everyone except me - I was the only person who had understood what she was going through, who understood what she had wanted and, sadly, understood what had to be done.

When she had tentatively mentioned these thoughts and intentions to her family they had all jumped back in horror and each one of them, without exception had said what most people would say

- No. Don't do it. We'll look after you. It will all be alright in the end.

As the words fell from their lips, Jemma decided to never tell them again, to make it seem as though it was just a passing thought, and to proceed with caution in order that they would be ignorant of her ultimate decision. She felt a certain disdain towards their formulaic reactions and responses, and their total inability to think about what she was going through, what she had to endure every day - what opinions and beliefs she held.

After her second attempt had failed, she was nearing her birthday; she would be thirty-four. She had become so determined to die that she felt she would never get to that age and the thought of enduring that day was a thought she tried to suppress; it was a milestone she did not want to reach. On more than one occasion she had mentioned to me that her family wanted to visit from Denver during that time and they were asking her what she might want as a gift. Then, one day she let it all flood out.

- I just want to tell them not to bother, not to waste their time. I want to scream down the phone that I will be dead by then anyway. I won't be here to accept any gifts from them and I don't want to see them or deal with their pity. I don't want to see anyone. Having to put on a brave face is the last thing I feel like doing. If they see me like this, then they will call me every day and they will try to make me feel better. I know they have the best of intentions, but I just don't care anymore. All I want is to be gone, and I want to be gone before I have to go through the charade of another birthday I don't want to acknowledge.

I was struck by the conviction with which she spoke about her death. I was shaken by the unwavering certainty of her words; she had made a decision that was, to her, irreversible and inevitable, and it seemed that she had also put a time constraint on her existence. Although we had spoken of this many times, she had never been quite so verbally combative about her intentions.

Her prophecy did not come true, she lived to see her thirty-fourth birthday; her family came to visit, but she only saw them once for an hour or so. She said she did not feel up to spending time with people - and they gracefully acknowledged her wishes.

For my part, I was uncertain as to what to do to 'celebrate' this birthday she did not want to acknowledge. If I asked her what she might like to do she simply brushed it aside as if it would never exist for her anyway, but as the day drew closer I knew I had to do something; to buy her a gift would almost insult her intentions, to not buy her a gift would perhaps make me come across as unloving.

After much deliberation, I decided to buy her favorite ice cream cake from Baskin Robbins, pumpkin flavored. I had it adorned with all of our favorite little sayings, I also bought her other treats that she could eat and enjoy, read and discard, but nothing permanent, only gifts that were 'disposable'. There was a melancholy that permeated throughout the day. Her disbelief at having reached this milestone, mixed with my knowledge at suspecting that this would be the last birthday we would ever share overwhelmed any joy we had at spending the day together; it was becoming increasingly difficult to know how to act and what to do when I was around her. I wanted to ease her troubled soul, to take her mind off the finality of her days, but I had to also respect the severity of her wishes and the consequences her actions would have on my life.

Once her birthday was "over and done with" she spent every single day of that following fortnight wishing for her final breath, wishing for her death. Now that she was so near the end of her journey, I was the one left to contemplate our lives together.

I would never be able to replace her, of that I was sure. Jemma was a special and unique person, someone whose words and actions lived together, who held strong opinions in a serene way, who did not deserve the hand she had been dealt, who suffered without anger or resentment.

It was only because she was so brave that I was able to carry out my side of our silent bargain. My pain at watching her as she had to endure such misery was the reason that I understood and supported her decision. A decision I could not and would not try to alter.

And with these thoughts, I allowed myself to pack up the booth at the end of the Sample Sale, and I drove myself home to Laguna, to my place on the beach, as if Jemma was with Christina and they were having a girl's weekend in Hollywood - that was the reason that Jemma had suggested for me to not have gone back to her place on the Saturday night. That was the alibi.

As the minutes went by, as the daylight faded, as her life hung in the balance and as I processed the information within me, I was learning to accept Jemma's death on her terms.

25

I arrived home and immediately went for a walk on the deserted winter beach. It was a sunny afternoon but the wind was strong and the whitecaps on the ocean were plentiful. Walking on the beach at this time of year was a way for me to sort through my thoughts and fears, a time of solitude to appreciate nature and to feel the coolness that emanated from the sea. It was usually a refreshing experience.

I remembered the last time Jemma had come here, to my little house with the ocean as a back yard. She had asked me to drive her through the canyons so she could perhaps drive off the cliff if the worst came to the worst and all other options ran out. We had been weaving through the mountain roads around Laguna trying to decide where she might be able to launch the car to her inevitable fiery death hundreds of feet below. I was driving her car and I was not at all enthusiastic about this approach to her demise - it seemed riddled with problems. We had stopped at every possible place looking for a clear, perpendicular cliff that would allow for the required plunge. It was unbelievable, but as I got out of the car and looked over the edge I expected to see a sheer drop below me - instead there was an angled mountainside covered in lush vegetation that would catch the car and leave her stranded, or would cushion the fall and leave her in agony with broken limbs but no finality.

After an hour or so of half-hearted looking, Jemma needed to use the bathroom. I gladly abandoned this morbid field trip and drove to my house; I helped her out of the car, passed the gate, through the front door, down the stairs and onto the toilet. Afterwards, I helped her back up the stairs and onto a deck chair over-looking the ocean. As we waited for the dolphins to come by, she spoke about her dreams and wishes should she have to come back to this world.

- If we do have to come back here, I hope I come back as a dolphin. We could be dolphins together, that would be good, hiding in the ocean.

We both agreed that coming back as a dolphin would be the perfect answer, to live in this world without dealing with human issues, in an ocean so vast that we could lose ourselves if we so desired, able to communicate without the need for words; a serene life, surrounded by beauty.

Years before, after we had returned from our trip to Hawaii, she had sent me a card with a pair of dolphin swimming side by side in crystal clear blue water. Inside the card she had written -

This is where we will meet in our next life...

How Angels Die - A Confession

Free at last!
I think it might be heaven.
xoxo

When we used to go kayaking on the weekends, Jemma would be so keen to see the dolphins that she was like a little child waiting for her birthday, yet, without fail, on the occasions that the dolphins did come by, she would suddenly go quiet because they were so close, so powerful and so imposing. She was in awe of them really, she respected and feared them in one way and wanted to hug them in another. It always used to make me smile to see her so overwhelmed and so full of joy.

A few years before, on a cold winter afternoon, we were on my deck watching the huge Pacific rollers crash on the beach below when we saw a pod of dolphins appear to our left. As we watched them, we could see the whole face of the wave exploding onto the sandy shore. All of a sudden, just as one wave was about to come thundering down, a dolphin came flying out of the back of the wall of water, flew twenty feet through the air and dove straight back into the sea - it was almost acrobatic in its agility, a lone missile shooting out of the sea spray and then back into the ocean beneath it - Jemma screamed as loud as she could and then she jumped up and down and began clapping her hands with the thrill of what we had seen. She hugged me and kissed me and held on to me as the dolphins continued to swim by - neither of us ever quite got over seeing that dolphin, it was almost magical, like a dream scene that nobody would ever believe. We talked about it often after that day and every time we did her eyes lit up with excitement and happiness.

On this occasion, her last time here, I was holding her hand and looking at her while she scanned the waves for a fin. I studied the stillness of her visage and then I saw a tear trickle down her face. She made no effort to wipe it away.

- What's the matter, Angel?

A moment later, without taking her eyes off the water, she replied, quietly

- I'm never going to see this again.

At that moment, as the words fell from her lips, I knew it was true - a chill ran through my whole body. She would never see this again. It was a monumental thing to comprehend, a comment that carried so much finality and so much despair. It was almost too much to deal with, too much for our minds or hearts to grasp. I held her hand that day as we watched the waves disperse along the shore, together by the ocean for the last time. And then, unexpectedly she turned to me and said

- Will you do it with me?

How Angels Die - A Confession

I was stunned into silence; I knew what she meant, I knew exactly what she was asking, but I feigned ignorance.

- Do what? - I asked.

She did not miss a beat with her reply.

- Die with me. We could leave together...

My heart dropped when she said this; my words of certainty over so many years coming back to haunt me yet again. I stalled. I looked away. She looked at me, waiting. The heat swelled into my cheeks.

- I don't know, Angel - I stammered - I don't know.

She was silent for a while. She did not need to speak for me to feel her disappointment. I did not need to look at her to feel a sense of duty rise up in me and then disappear, slowly bubbling away but bringing no relief to my sense of indignity. I was, after all, thirty-seven years old. This was my plan. To die. Instead, Jemma, My Angel, was taking my place.

I was shamed into silence. I was the one who had spoken of suicide so flippantly all those years ago; she had every right to think I would do it with her. The onus was on me. I had failed to keep my word - I would be punished for the rest of my life.

When she spoke again, she spoke with a sense of finality.

- When I'm gone, will you scatter my ashes in the ocean?

I paused, and then I replied, quietly.

- Yes... With my heart.

We never spoke of it again but I know that my sadness was compounded by letting her die alone. My heart ached at my weakness, my mind convincing me that I had done the right thing even as my thoughts wandered to what might have been.

I had no reason to die, I felt a responsibility to my mother, she had already suffered the loss of one child to a cruel twist of fate, and I was, for all intents and purposes fully healthy, but I felt a huge weight in my heart - a part of me wanted to honor the love that Jemma and I had, and that part of me wanted to leave with her, despite the pain I would cause my mother. In the end my survival instinct overrode my emotions, but not a day goes by when I do not think of being with Jemma again - what if? I ask myself. What if?

Now, as I walked along the sand with the wind on my face, tears fell from my eyes and I made no effort to wipe them away... I was never going to see her again - not in the way I would want to remember.

How Angels Die - A Confession

Each one of my footprints in the sand were washed away by the waves as I continued walking; like Jemma's life, once there, but now gone, just a memory, an illusion, a forgotten moment.

I kept on walking.

26

I would have to 'find' her at some stage, I thought; should I go tomorrow night or wait until Monday? I knew that she did not want a scene made over her death, she wanted to slip away quietly - she did not even want a funeral.

If I went on Sunday night everyone in the apartment complex would be home and it would be a commotion. Perhaps it would be better to go on Monday morning, but this meant that I had to wait longer and suffer more before I knew for certain that she had succeeded. It was a dilemma that had no right answer. If I arrived at the apartment too early then I might not give her enough time to pass away which would be her worst possible option; if I took too much time to discover her, then it might look suspicious as to why I had not gone before. I had to think of her first, I had to be sure that this time it had worked and she was released from this hell.

I decided to wait until Monday morning. It left me in purgatory, in a fog of unreality with only one thought on my mind - My Angel. My Sweet, Sweet Angel.

How Angels Die - A Confession

I was cold now, chilled, and so I walked off the beach and up the wooden steps to my beach house. Nobody was around on this cold, blustery day - I did not have to put on a brave face or make inane conversation. I washed the sand off my feet, opened the door and went inside. Now, all I could hear was the soft crashing of the waves through the closed French doors; my body began to move in slow motion as I switched on a single reading light and sat down in the armchair that faced the ocean.

The tide was out and the sun was fading, the clouds had taken on a pinkish hew and the sky behind was a soft, ice cold blue. I held in my hand a manila envelope with every card, note, fax and letter that Jemma had ever given or sent to me. I opened up the cards one by one, each filled with love, terms of affection, scribbles, kisses and hugs; some with lipstick imprints of her lips where she had kissed the card, others with little drawings and loving notes.

She used to send me faxes in the early days as if they were party invites. She would write the date, time and location, followed by the occasion, which was invariably 'for some kisses' or 'to give and receive loving'; I also had all the Birthday and Christmas cards she had sent me, the Thank You notes and the Love notes, the 'non-Valentines' cards (because we refused to celebrate such a ridiculous day, but did not want to forget how much we loved each other). She was brilliant at finding relevant and funny cards. Her words were always complimentary and loving.

How Angels Die - A Confession

As I read these messages, these memories, it dawned on me that those days had passed too, that my future would always incorporate the loss of one I loved so much. I would be marked by this, this tragedy, forever. I felt my stomach ache and I sensed my eyes well up with tears again.

I wondered how I would carry on, how I could contemplate a life without her in it, what joy would there be for me in my heart when this was shattering everything I knew to be good, true and honest. Jemma's love, our relationship, this life, were all intertwined for me. There was never a moment in seven years when I thought I would be without her for the rest of my life; she was such a loving, sweet, kind and understanding person.

She allowed me space and time, and every time, without fail, that she answered the phone - she did so with a smiling voice; whenever we saw each other our time was filled with affection. We were together for all the right reasons; there was no insecurity, no desperation, just pure admiration and respect. We each had our faults, but we were perfect for each other, we came together with the same opinions and beliefs, doubts and issues. We believed in love, but we celebrated the individual. We were supportive without smothering each other; we could explore the depths of our souls and our minds without becoming depressed. We were, ultimately realistic about life, the way it works, the futility of the human race and the relative insignificance of each of us. We were content and happy, we communicated and we loved. To lose all of this did not seem fair to me, and to expect to replace it seemed wrong. It was wrong, it was unbearable. Today, I was losing my emotional foundation to a disease that was unforgiving. I could see no way forward.

I felt extremely solitary; lost and alone. I ached in my heart and in my body. I read the words she had written so lovingly and so regularly, I read them over and over again as tears streamed down my face. I sobbed, my whole body lurching with the sadness, physically erupting with the grief, hollow with the loss. I was unable to stop myself and did not want to stop because it would mean creating some sort of distance from the situation and then I would be too far away from her.

I wanted to be with her. I did not want her to die, to disappear, to be just a memory and some cards. I wanted to cry, to feel her in my tears, to embrace her existence so that I would never have to let her go. This way, with tears as a reminder, at least I was close to her in my mind and I could feel that I had not lost her quite yet.

Sitting in my chair, in my small house in Laguna, as the monochrome dusk turned into a grey, dark and cold night, the ocean became the color of molten lead. I now tried to imagine her there in her quiet apartment - the darkness gradually enveloping each room, the lights all turned out. She was alone, lying in the bed, still, perhaps dead.

These thoughts broke my heart. Again.

I began to grieve. Again.

27

I knew I had to occupy myself over the next day or so - partly as an alibi, partly to make the time pass more rapidly and partly to corrupt my emotions into believing that life was carrying on as normal so I would not devastate myself into irreversible melancholy over the horrific reality.

As the first part of my alibi, I arranged to go for dinner in Santa Monica with some friends who were in Los Angeles visiting from England. I could not possibly bear the thought of being in Beverly Hills or Hollywood tonight; the proximity to Jemma's house would cause me too much distress and I would not be able to function with any semblance of normality, which was imperative if I was to have a believable story.

At this stage, I still had no idea how hard the police would review the last two days of Jemma's life. I had not dared to fully research the seriousness of what I was doing in the eyes of the law in case it held me back from being there for Jemma in the way she might need me. I had to be certain that anybody who saw me during that time would give a credible account of my behavior being completely normal in order for me to maintain ignorance as to her self-inflicted demise.

I managed to muster up the energy to have a shower; but as I thought about what to wear I was consumed by the insignificance of everything.

What did it matter what I wore, what car I drove, who my friends were, if I was loved, liked, or despised? It all boiled down to nothing anyway - Jemma was dying. Or dead. And nobody knew. Nobody was considering it in their daily routine; nobody was checking up on her and, even if they did, it made no difference now. She was gone. Everything she had ever done, every thought she ever had and every word she ever said was immaterial; it had all vanished with her last breath.

My love for her meant nothing now, except to me; to me it was total loss and total devastation, but that made no difference to anybody else. What did it matter what I did tonight? Or if I was accused of helping her commit suicide? It was her right to do as she wished, so as far as I was concerned I would be remiss not to support and love her to the very end.

As these thoughts bounced around in my head my mood darkened, only to lighten again in an instant of relative emotional control which would be followed by a plunge back into the abyss.

How Angels Die - A Confession

I drove up the 405 freeway and along the 10 West to Santa Monica. I was acutely aware I had to keep up appearances in order that My Angel had the time to pass on. I assumed by now, twelve hours later, she would have succumbed to the massive intake of sleeping pills. She would have faded away as her heart slowed to a pace that could no longer keep the breath flowing into her lungs. She would have dissipated to stillness.

However, I am a cautious person. I believe very strongly in being certain before taking action and I was conscious of the possibility that twelve hours might not be quite enough time for her body to completely collapse. If she was discovered now, the paramedics might be able to bring her back to life. It was imperative for her that I did not allow anyone to know that I had left her that morning, to die. I had made sure to double lock the door so that she would not be discovered until I deemed it the right time.

The only person who might come between Jemma and certain death was Christina, but she had been told the previous day that Jemma and I would be spending the weekend in Laguna. Recently, they were communicating daily by phone along with a visit once or twice a week. When we spent weekends in Laguna, Christina would not pester Jemma and so I figured that I had some time before having to worry about that scenario.

How Angels Die - A Confession

Once my friends and I had sat down to eat dinner at Lilly's on Abbot Kinney in Santa Monica, and the conversation began to flow, it became a little easier to give off an air of relaxed attentiveness. I tried my very best to concentrate on what was being said, to interject with the odd sarcastic comment, to laugh at the appropriate times and to eat as I normally would. None of my friends seemed to notice anything untoward. I was not too worried as I said my goodnights and climbed back into my car for the lonely and quiet drive home...

28

The night had passed slowly, painfully slowly; I had exhausted myself to a few moments of sleep in between the nightmarish visions and I awoke as the sun was beginning to crack open the sky over the ocean - colorless grays and blues that reflected my mood. I lay on my side facing the water as the daybreak loomed and the light of day unfurled across the horizon.

I felt dull with sadness. I was numb to my own existence, yet acutely aware that Jemma still lay undiscovered in her bed.

The thought of her, lying there, dead, alone, made my heart ache with anxiety and grief. I felt guilty for leaving her - I felt sick with myself and the world for allowing this to happen. It was wrong that she lay there, her body still, her soul departed, her life over, while I was still here, breathing, thinking, acting, reacting, able to see the sky, the ocean, the dolphins, the things that she would not see again; the sun still rose in the sky, the waves still reached the shore, the world turned. It made no difference, she was gone.

How Angels Die - A Confession

And I had left her to die.

It was too late now. I had accepted this path. I had to complete the task.

I pushed the covers back and got out of bed. It was 9AM. I wandered into the kitchen. I poured out some cereal, I cut up some fruit, I made a cup of coffee. This was my Sunday morning ritual...

Then, all of a sudden, my cell phone rang. I glanced at the screen and saw one word:

Angel.

29

I stared in disbelief at the word on the screen:

Angel.

Was it the police? Had they found her already? Should I answer?

I let it ring. I picked the phone up from the counter and just held it uselessly in my right hand. The ringing stopped. Silence. I watched the screen, waiting for the message icon to appear. A few seconds later it popped up in the top left hand corner - a small envelope. I pressed the voicemail button, waited for the connection and then I heard the monotone voice at the end of the line.

- You have one - new - message ... First - new - message.

My hands were weak as I held the phone to my ear. They shook ever so slightly. My heart was suspended in the intensity of the moment.

These were the words I heard:

How Angels Die - A Confession

- It's me... I woke up... What am I going to do?

Click. The line went dead. She had sounded faint, distant.

I called back immediately. The phone rang once, Jemma picked it up.

- Hi.

She sounded flat. Defeated.

- Angel? How do you feel? Are you okay?

- I feel groggy a bit. Angry. I'm very angry. Why didn't it work?

- I don't know, My Angel. I don't know. What do you want to do? What can I do? - I spoke quietly. My voice breaking with emotion.

I felt her pain and her anguish. This must have been hell on earth for her. This was hell on earth for her. My stomach was churning. We had said goodbye so many times, and every time it was more anxiety ridden, more acute, more difficult.

- I want to end it now. I want to do this before I cannot do it anymore. And I know I only have a few more days until I will be too weak. And then what will I do?

She was sure that soon she would not have the strength to even pull the trigger of the small handgun.

- Do you feel up to it? Are you sure? - I asked.

- Yes. I want to do it now. Should you come and check the gun, just in case?

- I don't know, Angel. I checked it the last time. I can come if you want, or you can try it and if it doesn't work I'll get it fixed. What do you think?

She spoke again. She sounded different.

- I'll try it. I don't want to do it this way, but I have no choice left anymore. And right now I'm so frustrated. This is the time.

- Okay, My Angel. I love you with all my heart. I love you.

- I love you too.

Still, I hoped that she might not go through with it. After the intensity of emotions I had felt last night, after the reprieve we had just been offered, yet again, I was left with just a glimmer of hope... But I was aware that I had to tread carefully so she would not see me as pressurizing her one way or the other.

- Angel?

- Yes.

- Are you sure you want to do this now?

- Yes. I'm sure.

- Okay... Okay. I love you, My Sweet Angel.

- I love you too...

I waited.

The phone clicked. I held it tight to my ear, I heard the line buzz and then go quiet. I looked at the screen. It read:

Angel. Disconnected.

30

As I stood looking at the ocean, I could no longer think about anything definitive. I would start a thought and then I would end it, or I would end a thought and instantly start another one; I was all over the place.

She had survived another attempt, perhaps it was just not meant to be. Perhaps she would recover in the end and we would resume our life as we had once known it.

I still held the phone in my hand waiting for it to ring. What was she doing now? Was she sitting on the bed, thinking about what to do next? Was she moving herself over to the bedside table, pulling out the gun, positioning herself with a pillow behind her head to catch the fatal speeding bullet, easing the gun into her mouth, the metal touching her teeth, her lips, her tongue... Silently counting to ten?

God - it was too brutal to even think about, to imagine her, weak and almost helpless as she held the small handgun, heavier than one might imagine, solid metal, cold and hard; her hand perhaps shaking, with tears trickling from the sides of her eyes down to her hair by her pretty ears, the short barrel pushed carefully to the roof of her mouth, as she slipped her finger onto the trigger, wavering, saying goodbye for one last time as her finger tentatively squeezed, the spring action taking over and then…

BANG!

That would be it. She would be gone in a second. Her body might shake for a moment before going completely limp; the gun still in her hand, her whole life over, meaningless.

Countless scenarios played in my head, but all of them seemed like fantasy, as if they were just ideas and none of them would actually happen. People do not just die like that I kept telling myself. One second here, the next gone.

In actual fact, they do. That is exactly how it is. This is why death is so difficult to deal with. Even when we know it is coming, we are still riddled with numerous conflicting and inexplicable emotions - guilt, anger, fear, sadness, loss, confusion. Yet, none of these words explain what was going through my heart and my mind on that Sunday morning as I stared aimlessly away from Hollywood and Laguna and out to sea.

I was numb, I know that. I was also tearful, the tears told me that. But I was not sure why. I do not think I felt guilt, although I wish I had been there with her, to at least soothe her, assure her, accompany her.

I felt frustration at not knowing what was happening, at not being allowed to help her because of the consequences. I was left in a dreadful dichotomy, this strange sense of wrong for wanting her to achieve peace aligned with this terrible fear of losing her.

There was no solution to this tragedy, only a conclusion; yet I did not know what that conclusion would be or when it might occur. And when that conclusion was reached, I had no idea how I would react, how I would live with myself for participating in something so final - how I would forgive myself for letting her die alone.

I paced a little to keep my legs from shaking. I think what I mostly felt was disconnected. The world was going about its business and getting on with life, My Angel was ending hers, and I was doing nothing.

Just waiting.

31

The phone I held in my hand did not ring again, although I kept looking at it to see if it would, or to try to will it to connect me to My Angel just one more time.

After a while, I decided I had better do something during the day to provide a credible alibi for myself if I was going to be safe from speculation when I found Jemma. For, despite the grief I was beginning to feel, I knew I had to be practical.

Yet, I sat there, devastated by the thought of her, My Angel, weakly reaching for the gun, contemplating the finality of her movements. I wondered if she would even have the strength to handle the kick back as she pulled the trigger. She was incredibly fragile now anyway; her body free-falling every day. The strength in her hands was fading as the minutes passed, and now, after having slept for over twenty-four hours, after having consumed so many sleeping pills, she would be even weaker, giving herself even less of a chance of completing this horrific task.

She had not cried when she swallowed the pills - if she had I could have held her. She was not angry - if she was I could have been angry alongside her. She was calm. She gave me nothing to cling onto before she had fallen asleep. Her movements had been deliberate in those moments. Thoughtless. Physical. Not emotional. I just hoped she could do what she had decided to do. I hoped that she would succeed in finding her nirvana.

I was not able to eat breakfast, I had no appetite. The healthy fruit and cereal sat in the bowl. The coffee stayed in the cup, half finished, cold.

I looked down at my phone. Lighter than a gun.

I scrolled through the names. Aimlessly.

Alibi. Alibi.

Cindy - an old friend, but not a close friend. Perfect. I knew she would not pry into my personal life - it was of no interest to her. She was a workaholic so we mainly talked business. I called. She picked up, happy to hear from me. I asked her if she wanted to go bicycle riding on the Huntington Beach pathways with me for the afternoon. She readily agreed and we arranged to meet up by the pier where we could rent some bicycles and ride around the area.

On the way from Laguna to Huntington I expected my phone to ring - Jemma. But no. It was silent. I could not sense what was going on. I thought she might have put the phone down after we spoke and decided to just get on with it. She had seemed determined to get it over and done with - perhaps this was a good attitude for her at this time. She could have done it within five minutes of us saying goodbye. Or she could be lying on the sofa, watching a TV show, deciding to do it later, when her neighbors were out. I did not know. And I could not find out. It was the not-knowing that made it so very difficult to deal with.

On the ride around Huntington, Cindy and I did not talk all that much; I was careful to cycle just far enough ahead or behind so that conversation was scarce. I was in no mood to talk about the mundane things in life and had no possible way of talking about what was going on in my head without implicating her in all that was going on in my world.

The sporadic conversation I did make as we rode our bicycles was usual for me. Jokes here and there, comments on passers-by, observations on the places and things we saw, easy words to make myself feel a little engaged with the world, to let Cindy know I was 'normal'. We did not stop for coffee or to eat. We just rode around at a leisurely pace. It was a warm day, a day in November to be remembered, despite the reason, or perhaps because of it.

I knew that I had to be perceived as unaware of what I was going to discover tomorrow. I was certainly not about to give the game away now. It was too late. The majority of people, should they hear someone was going to commit suicide and then, should they know of the location, would instinctively try to stop that person. They would think they were 'saving' them, 'saving them from themselves', doing the 'right thing', following the letter of the law, placing themselves in a moral position where human life is above all, sacred. But, in actual fact this act of being a savior would be thwarting someone's final wish - interfering with another's life (or death) - imposing their will upon another.

It is my belief that we have no right to stop someone harming themselves - we can surely advise against it, or try to help them should they seek our help, we can teach that it is against God's will, or against the will of nature, but we cannot and should not do anything to physically stop a suicide-in-progress; for the will and the energy and the forethought it requires to mentally prepare oneself for the final outcome is unimaginable to many of us.

Therefore, I do not see suicide as a weak choice, I see it as another choice, in many cases the best choice, and often times the bravest choice.

We will all die someday, let us choose when that day should be if we wish. We are in control of very little in this life, least of all when it shall end, so, should this life become unbearable, whether mentally, physically or both, then why would we conclude that it should be continued at any price?

How Angels Die - A Confession

I am not sure how successful I was at acting normally around Cindy. She made no comments as to my well-being. I can safely assume that I played my part with distinction and she was none the wiser. At any rate, we returned the bicycles a couple of hours later. We departed and went in opposite directions. She had work and I had receipts to garner in order for my alibi to be secure.

I drove back to Laguna, passed my house and into the maze of streets where there are stores, coffee shops, restaurants, a playground for children, and other businesses that entice one to linger aimlessly. My mission was to have proof I was nowhere near Jemma when she committed suicide; despite it being all I really wanted, to be by her side, to hold her and to love her as she moved on. This society did not give me that choice, it left me no choice. If I was present at her suicide, I was certain to be arrested. I had to account for my whereabouts at the time of her death.

Dutifully, I went to the Coffee Bean & Tea Leaf. I stood in line, and ordered my usual - a Caramel Latte. I walked to the benches that encircle the playground where kids gather. I watched the parents or nannies play repetitious games demanded by young children. I used to joke with Jemma that I came here to remind myself of why I did not have kids. The screams and laughter, the screams of laughter, the chatter, the pitter patter, the slight squeaking of the swings and the rustle of paper from takeout meals all served to pre-occupy my mind as I sat there, sipping my hot coffee in the warm, low, winter sun.

I was happy not to talk, not to see anyone I knew, not to have to 'fake it'. An hour must have passed before I took it upon myself to move, to walk to a trash can and deposit the empty paper coffee cup.

It was, by now, three o'clock or so. The afternoon light was fading. I decided to peruse a few of the shops so people would see me. I could always use this as extra proof I was nowhere near Hollywood. I bought a candle from one of the stores to space out my receipts. I said a quick hello to my friends in another store and I withdrew some money from the bank. I kept my profile as high as I could bear and then I climbed back into my car and drove home.

Five minutes later I was opening the door to my little haven, away from prying eyes. As I set down my car keys and organized my thoughts, I picked up my home telephone and I called my mother in England. It was past eleven o'clock at night there, but I knew she would be awake.

- Hi, Mum.

- Hello. Darling. How are you?

The tears fell straight away and I sobbed quietly.

- Not very good - I said.

How Angels Die - A Confession

- What's the matter, darling? Is it Jemma?

- Yes. I think she might have done it. But I don't know. And I can't go there, not yet anyway.

I told my mother what had happened, what Jemma and I had done, what had failed, what was said, what Jemma might have accomplished. I told her that I was waiting - waiting until tomorrow morning to go to the apartment in Hollywood to find her. Other than that I was helpless.

I felt for my mother as the words left me - to hear your only remaining son crying hopelessly and talking aimlessly about the person he loved - being six thousand miles away and unable to do anything other than listen must have been heart-breaking and worrying for her. But I think she would have rather known than to have later found out what I went through without having been there for me on some level.

She knew of Jemma's plans; she was aware of the situation without knowing too many details and to her credit, she never imposed a negative edict onto the information I gave. She was concerned, naturally, for Jemma, for me, but she always listened objectively and helped me to justify my emotions. She was as a mother should be - supportive, loving and kind. She did not judge. She simply listened and responded. There was nothing more she could do for me.

We talked for a while. As we talked I became more calm and more reasoned. Part of me, the part filled with hopelessness, accepted death as the inevitable; the other part of me, the part that had been nurtured by the society we live in, was devastated by the idea of losing Jemma - the manner of her death, the details that I could not quite accept no matter how many times I tried to imagine them.

Talking it through with someone who was non-judgmental was what I needed. My mother, a bereavement counselor, was, as always, amazing. As the minutes passed, I was able to control my raw emotions. I finally allowed myself to accept the irreversible. I became more calm but no more settled.

Mum told me to call whenever I wanted. She had done all she could for now. We said our goodnights and I remained hollow, in the chair, facing the setting sun.

There must have been a moment when it happened, I thought; the moment when she pulled the trigger - the moment when she left. What was I doing? Was I standing looking out to sea? Or riding a bicycle? Or driving my car? What was I doing and why didn't I feel or sense it?

I lit the candle I had bought earlier in the day. A flicker of light for Jemma.

How Angels Die - A Confession

I sat staring at the ocean, scanning the waves, waiting for the dolphins to swim by.

But there were no dolphins this evening.

32

I existed now, dulled, to the point where I drifted in and out of consciousness. I would come back around as if I had been sleeping, but my eyes were open the whole time. My mouth was dry, my mind was empty. I was trance-like. Vacant.

My breathing had also become labored. I could not draw in deep breaths and every so often I would feel like I did not have enough air to make it to the next minute. It was not worrying, just a little odd. My chest would heave until I grabbed enough oxygen to satisfy my lungs, during which time I would take shorter breaths to simply survive. This method of breathing became normal after a few hours.

I was anxious. I did not know for certain that Jemma was gone, but if I took an educated guess I would say that she most likely was. Shivers ran through my entire body as that truth was repeated over and over in my mind.

I did not know what to do. I waited for time to pass. The candle glowed softly as the day faded.

How Angels Die - A Confession

At six o'clock I picked up my home phone. I punched out Jemma's number. I put the phone back down. I wanted to call, but what if she picked up?

Worse still, what if she didn't?

I stared blankly.

I picked up the phone again and I hit redial.

I heard the ringing. Click. The voicemail picked up. It was an automated voice, which made it easier to cope with. I left a message.

- Hi, My Angel. I hope you're having fun with Christina. Call me when you can. I love you.

I put the phone down.

She had not picked up. Perhaps she would call back.

I waited.

I was motionless. I was emotionless.

I was not there. I was elsewhere. I was nowhere.

Three hours passed by unnoticed.

It was 9PM. Dark. Cold. Blank. I had not even turned on the lights. I came back around, slowly. The candle still cast its subdued light. Shadows on the walls as the flame flickered.

I picked up the phone. I hit redial.

The automated voicemail.

I left a message. I think.

33

Nothing can prepare you for death. Not even knowing it will happen - not even knowing when and where and by what means - which almost makes it worse.

Perhaps the not knowing, the shock factor, actually helps us to cope with this one certainty in life. Perhaps the sudden and unexpected information of a death temporarily shuts down our system so we can handle the situation a little better, creating a mental disconnect or a padding that absorbs some of the anguish and softens the blow.

There was no shock for me.

Just the reality of knowing.

Tomorrow morning, I would be faced with death. Of that I had little doubt. Tonight I was faced with nothingness. There was nothing I could do. There was nothing I could say. There was nothing.

I suddenly felt scared and vulnerable. I was worried that I should not be alone tonight. I imagined the night on my own, the thoughts I would have to endure, the noises I would hear, the dreams I might have, the images I would conjure up. I also imagined that it would look suspicious if my alibi consisted of

- I was at home. Alone.

I called Cindy and asked if she had had dinner - I needed to be occupied, I needed to be distracted - she said she had not as she was still working. We agreed to meet for sushi near her house in an hour.

As I drove away from my home and towards Hollywood, it dawned on me that it was Sunday night and most restaurants close by 10PM. I called the sushi place and arranged to collect a takeout meal. I then called Cindy and suggested that I would bring the food to her place up in the Hollywood Hills. She agreed.

I was there by half past ten. We ate as we watched TV. We talked a little, mostly about her day, her work, the trade show she had to go to in New York on Tuesday. I made effortless conversation, aware that I was eight minutes from where Jemma probably lay, still, dead. It gave me chills to think about it, it upset me to be so close to her without being able to go there, but I still asked Cindy if I could stay over. I would leave early for the gym, I said. She said that was fine.

I went into the spare room at Cindy's house and I climbed into bed. I did not fall into sleep easily although my mind was surprisingly calm. I had managed to use up three hours of the night by leaving my house and coming into Hollywood; I was exhausted from the effort. My breathing was still labored. My anxiety increased. My mental processing was at once racing and blank. My heart was confused by the prospect of being shattered when the truth finally revealed itself in the harsh light of day.

Before I went to sleep, I thought about My Angel, My Sweet Angel, My Brave Little Angel. I knew she must be dead by now, she had not called; I sensed the lack of communication to mean only one thing. Her body would be lying there in her dark apartment with stillness and death lingering in the air.

I wondered if she was watching me now, waiting for me to find her. I wondered if she would see me find her, or if she would not want to see me suffer and would have left this world behind for the living to worry about. If she had done it, with a handgun, in her mouth, through her brain, I thought about her bravery - how brave she was to have finally carried out what so many think of and are tempted by, and so few succeed in accomplishing.

Too many times suicide attempts are viewed as a cry for help or attention. I knew My Angel did not want help, other than the emotional help and the physical help required to carry out her final wish.

How Angels Die - A Confession

The enormity of her strength made me shudder as I imagined that last split second before she pulled the trigger, before everything went dark.

I drifted... I slept... I woke up before the sunrise was complete. I got up and I dressed in my workout clothes. I walked quietly down the stairs and out of the door of Cindy's house, I climbed into my car and I started this final journey.

I arrived outside Jemma's apartment.

I turned off the engine. I did not get out of the car.

I sat there. I was completely empty, my mind was null and void; both my mental and my physical strength had left me.

I waited in my car for a long while before convincing myself that I had to confront reality.

34

I took one more step into the room and there she was.

My Angel was dead.

Lying on her back, diagonally across the bed, her hands by her side, the small handgun to her right, by her hip - the barrel was pointed towards her, which seemed wrong. Her face looked peaceful apart from the blood that was covering her bottom lip, her chin, her neck. It had seeped into the pillow and framed her whole head like a bloody halo. Her eyes were closed, her eyelids were pale, very pale. She was still. So still that it frightened me to go near her. I stood in the doorway. I looked in disbelief. I was in shock now - of that I was sure. I stepped cautiously to the end of the bed and I eventually spoke out loud to myself, and to her.

- You did it, My Angel. You did it... Oh, God... I miss you.

I did not cry yet. I stood there, my hand over my mouth in case I vomited, my eyes observing the scene. Her body was on the bed wearing yellow sweatpants and the white top she wore to sleep in, a sheet covered her torso, pulled over in a final act of modesty, her feet exposed, her hands by her side; blood, so much blood all around her head but nowhere else.

It was a macabre scene, her expressionless face, the stillness in the room, a vacuum, no noise, no movement. I could not even sense myself breathing.

Everything was still. So very still.

No smells. No sensations.

I blankly examined the bedside table with the clock, the empty wine glass, the phone that held my messages and had rung twice the night before when I called. I wondered how long she had been gone - how long she had been lying there. I wanted to touch her, to reach forward and put my hand on her foot, to have contact with her one last time, but I could not move forward. I was afraid I might disturb her, wake her, stop her on her journey although I knew she was gone.

I stood there, for a length of time I still cannot remember, staring, distraught, controlled, relieved, frightened. Disconnected. Completely disconnected from the scene laid out before me.

For a split second I considered touching the gun, turning it over so it faced away from her. It seemed to me that the gun pointing at her might implicate me in her death, it did not feel quite right that it would be pointing towards her if she had pulled the trigger and her hand had fallen away; I flicked through the possibilities in my mind, and then I decided not to touch anything.

I stood. Stock still. Sickened.

My phone was in my hand. I looked at it for a moment. Then I moved. I dialed 911.

- Emergency. How can I help you?

- I think my wife is dead. I just found her. I think it's suicide.

I do not clearly remember the rest of the conversation. She asked me for the address, the manner of suicide. She told me that the paramedics were on their way and that I should meet them at the front door. I put the phone down after I had thanked her. By now, I could no longer look at My Sweet Angel on the bed with all that blood. I turned, I left her in the bedroom, alone, I wandered into the sitting room and began walking in circles, I felt almost deranged with grief as I registered the enormity of what had befallen me, and her.

I sat down on the leather sofa, facing the road, looking through the sheer curtains at the cars passing by. It was rush hour. The rest of the world was on go. I had come to a full stop.

How Angels Die - A Confession

I was shaking, shaking from sadness, fear, confusion. I looked at my cell phone again. I dialed my mother in England. The phone rang, she picked it up.

- Hello?

- Mum? She's done it. She's dead.

And then the tears began to fall, my body released all of the anxiety and all of the worry that I had felt over the past two days. Months and years of bottled up fears were set free.

I was inconsolable, my tears were uncontrollable. Words were few and far between.

My mother was there, just there at the end of the line. She offered to fly out and see me if I wanted – if I needed. She let me cry and she soothed me as the sirens approached. When I saw the paramedics pull up outside the apartment complex I told her I had to go. I would call her when I could.

I left the apartment and walked towards the glass doors that separated the apartment complex from the street.

I opened one of the doors and let the paramedics into the outdoor foyer. I did not greet them verbally; I simply nodded and led them into the apartment, towards the corridor that went to the bedroom.

How Angels Die - A Confession

- She's in the bedroom on the left. Do I have to come in? I don't think I can look again.

They said it was okay for me to wait. Three of them walked passed me, noisily shuffling in their full emergency gear. They all looked at me, observed their surroundings, and kept walking without a word.

I sat back down on the edge of the sofa and I picked up the cushion that held Jemma's indentation. I knew that she was not mine anymore, the process of the law would take over, and she had been seen by others now, her privacy had been violated beyond anything she would have wanted. I could no longer protect her. I placed the cushion on my lap with the indentation facing me, the place where her head had rested so many times. I put my face on top and I cried - my body convulsing quietly.

A few minutes later, one of the paramedics left the bedroom and entered the sitting room. She stood there uneasily until I sensed her presence and turned towards her.

- There is nothing we can do. I'm sorry for your loss.

35

One uniformed police officer stood over me as I sat on the sofa; another was stationed by the front door. By now there must have been ten people in and out of the apartment. The paramedics had left, to be replaced by these two officers, two detectives and a coroner with his assistant. The officer standing over me refused to let me get a drink of water. Everything felt wrong. I felt uneasy.

These strangers now controlled the situation. They walked in and out of the apartment as if it was a hotel, they made callous comments on the scene as if I was not there; they asked me questions as if I was a criminal. They were, to put it mildly, doing their job. They would not allow me to make phone calls and they gave me only vague answers to any of my questions.

If I am fair, I must have looked like a suspect - cropped hair, stubble, sunglasses, tattoos. I held the square suede pillow on my lap, I looked straight ahead at the cars passing on the street outside, and every few minutes I let the tears stream down my face.

How Angels Die - A Confession

By this time I was having real trouble breathing, the breath would not catch in my lungs and so I had to pull the air in forcefully to feel that I was going to make it to the next breath. This symptom lasted for months as I grieved the loss of Jemma; it was a symptom of my sadness - of my devastation.

There was no sympathy on the faces of these strangers, just false words of condolence. One detective, a woman, asked me when I had last seen Jemma, why I came to the apartment this morning, whether I knew anything about the three empty bottles of sleeping pills in her bedside drawer, the bloodstains on the bathroom floor, or the bruises on her knees and elbows. I told her that Jemma had MS, that she fell often and without warning, that her life was becoming unbearable, that she had mentioned suicide, but only in passing, that she had often talked of wishing she could just fall asleep and never wake up.

The detective then informed me that there was a suicide note but she would not let me see it and would not tell me what was written. I asked her when she thought Jemma had passed, how quickly she would have died, whether she would have felt any pain? She did not know the answer to each of my questions. I asked if I could call Jemma's twin sister - she said it was best to wait. I asked her what would happen now - she said they were checking the scene, and after they had completed that task they would remove her body and then they would like to ask me some more questions.

I was left in limbo, purgatory. Again.

After two anguish-filled hours, they asked me to sit outside so they could begin an investigation and look through the apartment. The manager of the apartment complex, David, sat with me. He was calm and kind; he told me that Jemma was the first person he had rented to when he became the manager and that he had liked her very much. He also told me the detectives had asked him about me - he assured me he had told them I was a loving and devoted boyfriend. He, like everyone else, did not know we were married. As he talked, the coroner interrupted us to inform me that they would be removing Jemma's body soon so I should be prepared. He then gave me his card with Jemma's case number on it.

A few minutes later, the metal stretcher came out of the apartment, wheeled by two assistant coroners - laid out on the stretcher in a light green body bag was My Angel. They struggled through the doorway and down the three steps, the clanking and bumping made the movements very undignified. They talked as if they were moving a piece of furniture.

At least they talked quietly.

I remember staring vacantly as they passed. I was sitting down in one of the elaborate, white iron garden chairs by the pool. I wanted to stand - to pay my respects - but I was unable to move. I was numb, tears streaming from my eyes.

I no longer knew what to do or what to say. I bowed my head and sobbed.

Another detective came towards me, he fumbled in his pocket and then he gave me his card and told me to call him if I had any questions.

- I have one - I said - Did she feel any pain?

- No - He replied - She would have died almost instantly.

36

The female detective had asked me if I would mind being taken down to the police station to answer a few questions. I had agreed to go, even though I was overwhelmed and physically distraught by the scene I had witnessed just three hours before; a vision that I knew would haunt me for the rest of my life.

As I walked to the waiting patrol car, a sheriff to my left and the detective to my right, I could sense their distrust of me; their suspicion was obvious by the fact that they walked slightly behind me. I was aware that my emotional state must have been unnerving to them.

The sheriff said nothing more than

- Sir, please put your hands behind your back.

Our greatest fear had come true. I was suspected of something I did not do. As confused as I was by the request, I automatically did as I was told; my head bowed, my back hunched unnaturally, my arms slightly bent, my hands together just above my tailbone. I heard the click-click-click of the handcuffs and I felt the cold metal grip my wrists a little too tightly for someone who was innocent, who had endured a sight no human should ever have to see, especially when it was the one I loved more than any other.

Had I just confessed my guilt by allowing them to handcuff me? Was I now viewed as a murderer?

What had seemed like an innocent request had just turned into an accusation.

I was in serious trouble.

More than that, I was heartbroken.

I wished that I was dead too.

37

Once the handcuffs were secured, the officer put his hand on my head to protect it from bumping on the roof of the car as he guided me to sit in the hard black plastic rear seat. The detective then said

- You can take those off. He's not a suspect.

So, I was in the clear? They knew it was a suicide and not a murder?

I felt no relief whatsoever. I did not care anymore. I was functioning, but only just.

I called Christina - I was in the back of the squad car with the two officers listening.

- Hi, Christina.

- Hi.

- Are you sitting down? I need to tell you something.

- What's the matter? Is Jemma okay?

How Angels Die - A Confession

- No... I don't know how else to say this... She's dead.

- How? What happened?

- She shot herself. I found her this morning. They wouldn't let me call you before. I'm sorry.

- Shot herself? Where did she get the gun?

- We got it a while back. She was scared when I was out of town. She made me help her get it and told me not to tell anyone.

- Oh God.

- Do you want me to call your mother? I am on my way to the police station to answer some questions. But I can call her if you like.

- No. No. I better do it - She paused - Will you call me later?

- Yes. As soon as I can.

I could not tell her the full truth. I wanted to, but Jemma had made me promise not to. So, I kept my promise. I am sorry for that, but in those moments and in the following days and months, I had to protect myself from any misgivings that the law might have had with my role in Jemma's death. I told her, and I told the detective at the police station a version of the truth that was as confusing as the truth would have been. But it was the best I could do at the time.

I exonerated myself from blame as Jemma had told me to.

38

Two days later, on the Wednesday, I drove to the Coroner's Office for Los Angeles County. It was a nondescript building with a three level parking garage.

I walked through the concrete pathways and entered the lobby. I gave Jemma's name and her case number to the girl behind the glass. She told me to wait.

A few minutes passed before she appeared at another window and handed me a manila envelope.

- This should be everything - She said.

- Does it contain her suicide note?

It was all I cared about.

She looked at the list of items.

- Yes - She replied.

- Thank you.

I took the envelope, left the building and walked towards the nearest set of steps. I walked past a woman with a stroller, and then past a couple who were smoking.

It was a quiet area. Deathly quiet.

I sat down on the top step of the six steps and I leaned against the round metal handrail. I opened the envelope carefully and sorted through the ten or so documents inside. They were all official notes and diagrams from the coroner, apart from one - a crumpled piece of yellow paper, lined, 11 by 8. I pulled it out of the envelope and I looked at it. In scrawled handwriting it read -

My Sweet Baby,
I am truly sorry that you will have to deal with this.
But I can't live like this with absolutely no hope.
I feel like I have no other option.
You have been the most amazing person I have ever had in my life. You have put up with and done more than anyone should ever have to with me.
Thank you so much for being the most kind, selfless, generous and beautiful person I have ever known.
I love you so very much!
Love! Love! Love!
Angel

39

Jemma's ashes were scattered on a deserted beach in Southern California. The tide was out, the Santa Ana winds were blowing a warm breeze, and the sunset was endless. The wispy clouds above were filled with pinks, blues, reds and grays, and the dusk lingered as the moon rose and cast its glinting light over the darkened water.

We placed her ashes within a circle of lilies and left them there for the tide to wash away.

I visit the spot often and I always do the same thing - it is what I did that day, when I said farewell. I write in the sand, in our special code -

I ♥ ·

In my wallet, I carry a photograph. It is a black and white miniature we took in a photo booth when we first became lovers, I am kissing her cheek and she is smiling directly at the lens. They were happy times.

I think of her every day. I miss her, I miss our easy love.

How Angels Die - A Confession

I still wear her horse shoe ring on my finger.

Sometimes I shudder at the manner of her death, but I know that there was no other choice at the time. I console myself by realizing she is now free from the illness she so courageously endured.

I often wonder if my pain would be easier to comprehend had the pills worked; whether a drifting exit from this life would have been better than a cruel and brutal explosion.

EPILOGUE

It is hard to quantify a life, especially one that is ended without fanfare, without occasion. I do believe we could, if we only opened our minds a little, allow death to be an experience that is peaceful, tranquil and dignified, even in the darkest moments of its demise. Perhaps Jemma's story, her life, her illness and her suicide will open us up to a more understanding and less desperate view of someone's will to pass away. I hope so.

I do not feel her around me. I have dreamt of her once or twice. I like to think that she left this place and will never return. I know this world is too cruel for one so gentle and kind - so loving and brave. But, if life is a circle, and death follows the same pattern, I hope she comes back as a dolphin, as she always wished.

Whenever I see a dolphin, I see My Angel.

How Angels Die - A Confession

Guy Blews Bio

Guy Blews does his very best to disturb the comfortable, but more importantly to comfort the disturbed.

He is the author of "Marriage & How to Avoid It", "Realistic Relationships", and "Less Thing$ More Love".

He has appeared on numerous Television and Radio shows as either a visionary or a pariah.

www.GuyBlews.com

How Angels Die - A Confession

Credits

Editor: Michael Chabries

Editor: Jahnavi Newsom

Graphic Designer: Ian MacGillivray

Photo Credit: Moriah Diamond

Waldorf Publishing
2140 Hall Johnson Road
#102-113
Grapevine, Texas 76051

www.WaldorfPublishing.com